10649945

The New Low-Carb Way of Life

The New Low-Carb Way of Life

A Lifetime Program to Lose Weight and Radically Lower Cholesterol While Still Eating the Foods You Love (Including Chocolate)

Rob Thompson, M.D.
with Diane Stafford

M. Evans and Company, Inc.
New York

The information contained in this book is not intended to serve as a replacement for professional medical advice. Any use of the information in this book is at the reader's discretion. The author and publisher specifically disclaim any and all liability arising directly or indirectly from the use or application of any information contained in this book. A health-care professional should be consulted regarding your specific situation.

M. Evans and Company, Inc.
216 East 49th Street
New York, NY 10017

Library of Congress Cataloging-in-Publication Data

Thompson, Rob, 1945-
  The new low-carb way of life: a lifetime program to lose weight and radically lower cholesterol while still eating the foods you love— including chocolate / Rob Thompson, with Diane Stafford.
     p. cm.
  ISBN 1-59077-031-5 (hardcover)
  1. Low-carbohydrate diet. I. Stafford, Diane. II. Title.
  RM237.73.T468 2004
  613.2'83--dc22

                          2004001733

Typeset and designed by Evan Johnston

Printed in the United States of America

0 9 8 7 6 5 4 3 2 1

Dedicated to my editor/writer wife, Kathy,
without whose moral support, and editorial advice
this book wouldn't have been written.

CONTENTS

PART 2: SETTING UP A PROGRAM THAT WORKS FOR YOU

PART 3: CUSTOM-DESIGNING YOUR DIET TO YOUR METABOLISM

ACKNOWLEDGMENTS

I am deeply indebted to my agent, Elizabeth Frost-Knappman, for recognizing value in what I wrote and helping me develop my message. Invaluable also were the talents of PJ Dempsey, Senior Editor at M. Evans and Company, who helped polish the manuscript. I appreciate the many hours Diane Stafford spent helping me organize and revise the manuscript. Richard Marek's advice on tone and Lito Tejada-Flores's teachings on skiing helped me find my voice. I appreciate David Paul's editorial assistance in the book's early stages. Thanks also go to Burt Weissbourd and Ellen Taussig for taking the time to read what I wrote and provide encouragement and advice. Without the help of my office staff, Lisa Gierlinski, Nadine

Warner, and Charlene Brown, I wouldn't have had the time or energy to write this book.

INTRODUCTION

Whe I started practicing medicine twenty-five years ago, the mentality that dominated nutrition was "you are what you eat." We thought people got fat simply because they ate fat and accumulated cholesterol in their arteries because they ate cholesterol. For years, doctors tried to get patients to cut out fat and cholesterol, but it didn't seem to help. They just kept gaining weight and having heart attacks.

Then, in the 1990s, the field of preventive cardiology exploded when discoveries about metabolism and blood vessel disease turned old ideas upside down. Doctors found ways to prevent, even reverse, heart disease by changing the body-chemistry problems that caused it. Medical authors called this era a "sea change" or "new paradigm" in cardio-vascular medicine. It has been my privilege, as a cardiologist, to be at the interface of these new concepts with the lives of patients, and it has been an exciting experience.

Along with advances in knowledge about heart disease have come new insights into the causes and treatment of obesity. Of course, weight-loss claims based on outdated ideas and junk science continue to proliferate, which has obscured the progress that has been made. Nevertheless, using new knowledge about body chemistry, we now find it possible to pinpoint the metabolic flaws that lead to weight gain in most overweight people, which allows us to correct those conditions and facilitate weight loss more easily and dependably than ever.

Of course, success in losing weight still depends on moti-vation. People have a limited capacity to change, which means there's no room for wasted effort. However, once they discover the right strategy, they are often surprised how easy it is to shed pounds. The trick is in finding the right strate-gy, understanding it, and believing in it.

In the years I've practiced medicine, I have developed a sense of what people know, what they want to know, and what they can accomplish. People have to deal with weight problems, high cholesterol, and diabetes every day of their lives, but it is tragic how much wasted and counterproductive effort there is. It has been frustrating to me that there just isn't enough time in the day to convey to my patients the insight and knowledge I think they need. The information isn't hard to grasp, but it's too complicated to explain to patients in the course of a routine doctor's office visit.

The New Low-Carb Way of Life is the consultation of my dreams. It is what I would tell a patient who is frustrat-ed by failed attempts to lose weight and worried about future health problems, if I had all the time I needed to do the job right.

If you are like most of the people I talk to, you will find the ideas in this book enlightening. Having ideas that were formed by the media of recent decades, you may be astonished by the counterintuitiveness of some of the discoveries. My hope is that the insight you gain in reading The New Low-Carb Way will make your life easier and give you the edge you need to deal successfully with these sometimes stubborn but imminently curable problems.

PART I
GEARING UP
FOR THE NEW
LOW-CARB WAY

Part I explains how you can avoid diabetes and lose weight by abandoning pointless and frustrating "universal" diet plans, instead using a regimen that is based on your body's unique metabolizing traits. The cutting-edge information in the book's opening chapters deals with the following subjects:

▶ Brand-new developments in nutrition that drastically alter the weight-loss picture;
▶ Cholesterol demystified;
▶ How to work with (not against) your body's flawed mechanisms for processing cholesterol and carbs (if you have either or both problems);
▶ Why being fat is anything but jolly;

The New Low-Carb Way uses the unique approach of providing a personalized plan that's based on your own body chemistry and how it acts and reacts. This sets you on a clear-cut path toward pursuing and reaching your goals for healthier living: losing unwanted pounds, staving off diabetes, and preventing heart attacks and stroke.

CHAPTER I

Beyond Low Carb: Shining New Light on Dark Food Issues

I f you are like many people I talk to these days, you've heard about cholesterol and are concerned about it, but what really bothers you is your weight. You know being overweight is unhealthy, but mainly you don't like the way it looks and feels. It's a physical, social, and psychological encumbrance. And it just keeps creeping up. You've probably tried dieting, but that didn't work the way you hoped. You lost a few pounds, but it all came back. You know exercise helps, but you can't seem to muster the energy to do it. Chances are, you're a little discouraged.

You may also be getting a little worried. It was bad enough when your weight was just a matter of looks—now you're wondering if it could cause serious health problems. You know that being overweight raises your risk of heart disease and diabetes. Maybe your doctor told you that your "bad cholesterol" was high or your "good cholesterol" was low, or that your blood sugar was rising.

Everywhere you turn, you get hit with dietary advice. Every nutrition expert on the globe is hawking a new diet, and the funny thing is, they often contradict one another. Some weight gurus tell us to eat less fat and more carbohydrates; others recommend the opposite. Some advocate vegetarianism; others say we should eat more meat. So many weight-loss solutions are touted that you can't help but conclude the obvious: none of them works very well.

A LITTLE SKEPTICISM IS A GOOD THING

You need to be skeptical of things you hear and read about weight loss, because there's a lot of wackiness in the field of nutrition. Sensationalists and pseudo-experts comb the nooks and crannies of food research looking for tantalizing factoids, and then report them out of context as if these items represent the hottest news coming down the pike. They play on people's fascination with the notion that small amounts of potent, heretofore unrecognized substances in foods can cure or cause disease.

Furthermore, some diet-book authors encourage food extremism that has no basis in scientific fact. Claims that we're deficient in a particular vitamin, that hidden pollutants are making us sick, and so on, ignore the fact that researchers have spent billions of dollars and millions of hours trying to find links between diet and disease, and for the most part, have come up empty-handed. Remember, too, that when useful information is found, researchers are quick to spread the news to the medical community.

The Cognitive-Dissonance Tango

One reason food experts are so adamant in their opinions is what psychologists call *cognitive dissonance*. When people make a choice, they tend to seek out information that supports their decision and discount information that contradicts it. Avoiding contradictory information reduces inner conflict, or cognitive dissonance. If a person makes daily decisions to eat a particular way for years, that individual will invariably become convinced of the wisdom of such a regimen and see alternatives in an unfavorable light.

Indeed, most diet gurus try to eat the way they preach. Eating is a highly personal activity. If these people changed their opinions, they would have to admit not only that their ideas and statements were off-base, but also that they were consuming the wrong food. It would create too much cognitive dissonance.

The Human Body Is Adaptable

Another reason experts can't agree on what constitutes a good diet is that it's difficult to detect concrete differences in people's health based on what they eat. Our bodies have an amazing capacity to take what we eat, convert it to what our bodies need, and get rid of the rest. Nutritionists may nitpick about the fine points, but human beings generally do well on any kind of diet as long as it contains some plants and some animal products.

Fortunately for us, in recent decades, scientists have acquired some important lessons on the ways in which unbalanced diets result in obesity, diabetes, and heart disease. At the same time, though, because these discoveries contradict previous notions that people held dear, the new ideas have created heated controversy.

So, if you're skeptical of weight-loss claims, you have good reason to be. Despite all the dietary advice peddled in the media today, Americans just keep getting fatter. That makes it abundantly clear that if an answer exists, it has eluded many of us.

For that reason, it's important to tell you that the advice I give here is based not only on my interpretation of medical research, but also on the experience I've accumulated in twenty-five years of practicing preventive cardiology. I have seen the strategies I advocate help people lose weight, lower cholesterol, and prevent diabetes. The newest concepts about nutrition have bolstered my confidence in these approaches and inspired me to share them with you in this book.

OVERTURNING LONG-HELD BELIEFS

The good news is that science is coming to the rescue. In the last couple of decades, billions of dollars have been spent on research into human metabolism, and the investment is finally starting to pay off. Scientists have made remarkable breakthroughs in their understanding of the way lifestyle and genetics interact to influence such things as weight and cholesterol. This new knowledge has overturned many of the notions doctors and nutritionists took for granted for years, and at last, new, more effective ways of losing weight, lowering cholesterol, and preventing diabetes are emerging.

Seeing the Proof Up Close and Personal

As a preventive cardiologist who has spent more than two decades specializing in treating conditions that lead to heart and artery disease, including obesity, high blood pressure, high cholesterol, and diabetes, I have grown as familiar with my patients' weight fluctuations and blood tests as I have with their faces. In a clinic equipped with analyzers that quickly measure blood levels of good and bad cholesterol, triglycerides, and glucose, I have observed the responses of thousands of people's weight, cholesterol, and blood glucose to assorted lifestyle changes and medical interventions.

In the past few years, largely owing to discoveries about human metabolism, my approach to helping people with weight problems, high cholesterol, and diabetes has evolved in ways I could never have predicted even a decade ago. Perhaps the most surprising turnaround has been in my thinking about diet.

Dr. Atkins Was Right

Today, understanding what I now know to be true, I have a newfound respect for the wisdom of another cardiologist, the late Dr. Robert Atkins. In the 1970s, Atkins popularized a weight-loss diet in which he advocated almost completely eliminating carbohydrates such as fruit, vegetables, and grains but continuing the consumption of fatty foods, including eggs, meat, butter, and cheese. The diet helped people lose weight but fell into disrepute because it encouraged them to eat cholesterol-containing foods at a time when doctors thought dietary cholesterol was the main cause of heart disease. However, in recent years, many of Atkins's critics have come to realize that they should have listened more closely to what he had to say.

New studies have confirmed what Atkins contended all along: low-carbohydrate diets are more effective than low-fat diets for losing weight. And, dietary cholesterol is not nearly as harmful as the medical establishment thought.

Beyond Atkins

Although Atkins proved to the world that low-carbohydrate diets work and usually don't raise blood cholesterol levels, much has been learned about nutrition and weight loss since he first popularized his diet. Here are some examples of new concepts that are changing the way nutritionists and doctors think about obesity and high cholesterol:

▶ You probably don't metabolize nutrients the same way that your coworker or mate or neighbor does. People vary significantly in this respect, making a one-size-fits-all diet obsolete.

▶ Your body handles some carbohydrates differently than others. Now scientists can rate the effects of various carbohydrates according to how much they raise blood-glucose levels. Knowing the glucose-raising effects of various carbohydrates (see chapters 10 and 11) makes carbohydrate restriction easier, healthier, and more effective.

▶ You can tailor your diet, exercise, and medication to fit your particular body-chemistry type by taking into account certain details from your medical history and the results of a few simple blood tests. Small changes, crafted in that way, produce better results with less effort.

▶ You don't have to sneak sugar in the dark of night when no one's looking. It turns out that sugar, formerly the most guilt-provoking of foods, isn't the culprit. In fact, you can put sugar to good use to help you lose weight, lower your cholesterol, and prevent diabetes (see "Make Sugar Your Ally," chapter 11).

▶ You don't have to jog to tune up your body chemistry. You can use new concepts of muscle physiology to help make your metabolism hum like a long-distance runner's without your having to do all the huffing and puffing.

▶ You can benefit from effective medications for treating metabolic problems that weren't available when Atkins first popularized his diet. The very existence of these drugs changes the roles of diet and exercise in losing weight, lowering cholesterol, and preventing diabetes.

▶ If you truly have high blood cholesterol, it does little good to lower it a few percentage points. To decrease your risk of heart disease, *you have to slash it by a third to a half*, which usually requires cholesterol-lowering medication.

How the New Low-Carb Way Impacts Lives

I have developed a method of combining the scientifically validated elements of the Atkins diet with newer concepts of metabolism. This isn't just a diet; it's a way of finding the right strategy for each individual. The results have been amazing:

1. I see more people than ever shedding pounds and keeping them off without having to feel deprived or inconvenienced.

2. I see lower cholesterol counts than ever before.

3. I see people embrace the New Low-Carb Way with confidence. Having finally found the right strategy, they

know they have a way of losing weight they can stick with for life.

4. I rarely have to rush to the hospital to take care of someone with a heart attack. It hardly ever happens anymore! (When I first started practicing cardiology, this was a frequent occurrence.)

5. I know from experience that this approach is a path that people can follow, even if they aren't endowed with unusual willpower. Because I'm a practicing doctor—and not a diet guru—it's not good enough for me to tell people what they *ought* to do; I have to figure out what they *can* do. I assure you, *this is something you can do.*

GETTING HEALTHY THE NEW LOW-CARB WAY

Nutritional scientists have learned that what's making so many of us fat and diabetic isn't the tasty parts of our diet, or the pleasant textures, or the things that contain vitamins, minerals, and fiber. The real villain is a flavorless paste that has no nutritional value whatsoever—that relatively recent addition to our diets commonly known as *starch*. Because we are physically and economically addicted to this substance, we eat hundreds of times more than our thinner, less diabetic ancestors did. The New Low-Carb Way will help you stop the damage. Tame this beast, and everything else—losing weight, lowering cholesterol, reducing your risk of diabetes—becomes much easier.

You can use new discoveries about body chemistry to tailor

your diet, exercise regimen, and medical treatment to your individual metabolism in ways that will give you the best results for your efforts. With the right strategy in hand, you will be amazed how easy it is to accomplish what you set out to do.

You will discover that the New Low-Carb Way means you can get healthier by eating satisfying amounts of good food. It's absolutely true—you really can radically lower your blood cholesterol level, attain a healthy body weight, and prevent diabetes, yet still eat the foods you love, including chocolate, in satisfying quantities.

HOW THE NEW LOW-CARB WAY IS DIFFERENT FROM ALL THE REST

Although other popular diet books advocate low-carbohydrate diets—including *Dr. Atkins' New Diet Revolution*; *The South Beach Diet*, by Arthur Agatston, M.D.; and *The Zone*, by Barry Sears—The New Low-Carb Way is different in several important ways.

1. It teaches principles. Once you understand how your body handles nutrients and what causes people to gain weight and develop heart disease, you won't need the kind of list of day-by-day instructions the other books provide. You'll know automatically what you need to do.

2. It eliminates fewer foods. The New Low-Carb Way focuses on alleviating the harmful effects of only a handful of foods, not just by eliminating them from your diet but also by making your body better able to handle them when you do eat them. This is a key difference.

3. It advocates a personalized approach. Most diet books tout one-size-fits-all regimens, but the New Low-Carb Way shows you how to individualize your strategy. You learn how to profile your own unique metabolism by using details from your medical history, body measurements, and the results of a few simple blood tests, which you may already have on hand. This allows you to match your strategies for diet, exercise, and medication to your body-chemistry type. The upshot? A personalized plan that makes losing weight and lowering cholesterol much easier and more effective.

4. It blends with modern medicine. Many popular diet books pander to people's desire to avoid drugs by regarding medication as a last resort when diet fails. But the very existence of effective new medications for improving body chemistry changes the way you should approach diet and exercise from the start. The New Low-Carb Way is not a method for avoiding pills; it's a synthesis of diet, exercise, and medical strategies.

5. It focuses on healthy arteries. Excess body fat, cholesterol, and diabetes all lead to trouble the same way—by damaging arteries. Part 5 gives you a clear idea of what causes blocked arteries and what you need to do to keep your arteries healthy. Even if your primary interest is losing weight, you can direct your resources toward losing weight more efficiently if you don't have to worry about your arteries.

HOW TO USE THIS BOOK

To make this book work for you and your personal status in regard to cholesterol, weight, and general health, you should first read part 1 in order to understand the following principles of the New Low-Carb Way:

▸ What medical conditions are most likely to threaten your health and well-being

▸ What makes people overweight

▸ What is causing the current epidemics of obesity and diabetes

▸ What insulin resistance is

▸ What cholesterol is and how it affects your arteries

▸ How diet and genes influence cholesterol

Or, if you want to cut to the chase, start with part 2, which tells you how to determine your own body-chemistry specifics (the crux of the New Low-Carb Way), and then you can move on to the eating plan, outlined in part 3. If your chief interest is losing weight, read parts 1, 2, 3, and 4. If you mainly want to prevent heart disease or stroke, read part 1 and then skip to part 5. To give you a global perspective, here are the basics of the program I have devised:

Step 1 Gather information about yourself (parts 1 and 2). Obtain at least rough estimates of the items in the following list (the first three come from the results of your most recent blood tests). Chapter 3 tells you to use the information.

▸ Good and bad cholesterol levels

▸ Triglyceride level

▸ Blood glucose level

▸ Waist and hip measurements

▸ Family health history

Step 2 Profile your body chemistry. Use chapters 6 and 7 to uncover the answers to the following questions:

▸ Does your body have trouble removing cholesterol from your blood?

▸ Does your body have difficulty handling carbohydrates?

Step 3 Choose a strategy based on your goals and body chemistry. Use chapter 8 to help you zero in on one of the following:

▸ A strategy to help you improve your carbohydrate metabolism

▸ A strategy to reduce your blood cholesterol level

▸ A strategy for doing both

Step 4 Take action. After you choose your strategy, use the tools you need from the following list in order to achieve your goals.

▶ Reduce your intake of high-glucose-shock foods to eliminate glucose shocks (see chapters 10 and 11).

▶ Maintain a sensible fat intake to allow dietary variety (see chapter 12).

▶ Reduce bad fat to lower your cholesterol (see chapter 12).

▶ Reactivate muscle metabolism to relieve insulin resistance (see chapters 14 and 15).

▶ With your doctor's help, determine whether you need cholesterol-lowering medication (see chapter 18).

As you read this book, you will be pleased to discover that the New Low-Carb Way is really easy to do and definitely isn't about extreme food deprivation or exercise overkill. You just have to alter a few lifestyle habits, which will lead you to exactly what you want: weight loss, a healthier heart, and improved overall health.

KEY IDEAS FOR TAKEOUT

- In the past decade, new discoveries have turned old concepts about nutrition upside down.

- New and effective methods for losing weight, lowering cholesterol, and preventing diabetes are replacing old approaches.

- Researchers have found that dietary fat and cholesterol aren't as harmful, nor carbohydrates as harmless, as previously thought.

- It is now possible to pinpoint metabolic flaws that lead to weight gain and diabetes in most overweight people.

- The New Low-Carb Way will show you how to profile your body chemistry and tailor your diet, exercise, and medication to your particular body-chemistry type. This makes losing weight, lowering cholesterol, and preventing diabetes easier than ever.

CHAPTER 2

Syndrome X: Why I Changed from a Crusader Against Cholesterol to a Starch Buster

A low-carbohydrate, liberalized-fat approach may not make sense at first, but after you understand the rationale behind it, you will see why it makes perfect sense for most people trying to lose weight or lower cholesterol—not *all*, but most. First, let me explain how my own thinking about diet and metabolism has evolved over the past few years, and you will see how I, a traditionally trained, board-certified cardiologist, was converted. I went from advocating low-cholesterol, *high*-carbohydrate diets to a complete turnaround in attitude.

GROWING MY CHOLESTEROL KNOWLEDGE

In 1994, if you had asked me to recommend a healthy diet, I would have told you to cut down on cholesterol-containing foods like red meat, eggs, and dairy products and eat more carbohydrates—fruits, vegetables, grains, and starches. That was the standard low-fat, low-cholesterol diet that most doctors and nutritionists recommended for losing weight and reducing blood cholesterol levels.

I had heard of the Atkins Diet, which was popular in the early 1970s, but it sounded like a bad idea to me. How could an eating plan that allows so many meat and dairy products be good for you? And why cut carbohydrates? They're cholesterol-free. I figured Dr. Atkins was just old-fashioned. He started down that path before the public became aware of the dangers of cholesterol. I remembered when he was called before a congressional subcommittee to defend his methods and was publicly derided.

A decade ago, not many people remembered the Atkins Diet. I didn't know any doctors who recommended it. However, I remember a patient I saw in my clinic about that time who had scheduled an appointment with me because he had been on the Atkins Diet and wanted to be sure it hadn't raised his cholesterol level too much. He chose the diet not because he was ahead of his time; rather, he remembered it from the 1970s. (I suspect that he owned an old copy of Atkins's first book.)

It was obvious that he had lost a lot of weight. He described a diet full of red meat, eggs, and dairy products, but when I checked his blood, I was surprised to find that his cholesterol level was lower than ever. I remember thinking that was a little odd, but, truthfully, I didn't pay much attention to it at the time.

Since then, I have experienced a major change in attitude about diet. I have come to believe that for most people, the best approach for preventing heart and blood vessel disease is a low-carbohydrate eating pattern with moderate amounts of fat and protein. The main impetus to my conversion was the discovery of something called Syndrome X (see below). But first, let me explain how changes in my attitude about several other things set the stage for this transformation.

RETHINKING DIET

The longer I practiced medicine, the more I appreciated how frustrating and heartbreaking the problem of excess body fat was and how many health problems it caused. Besides being cosmetically unappealing, obesity had become a major risk factor for heart and blood vessel disease, but doctors treated it more as a lifestyle issue than a disease. Ten years ago, medicine had little to offer people who were overweight.

Addressing the Diabetes Issue

One thing that struck me as clumsy back then was the dietary recommendations that were given to newly diagnosed diabetics. You might call it the "diabetic U-turn." Before they developed diabetes, we would tell these folks (as we told all of our patients) that to lose weight, they should limit fat and cholesterol and eat more carbohydrates. But after they became diabetic, they quickly found out that starch and sugar drove their blood sugar up while fat and cholesterol had little effect on it.

You may think that the best and easiest advice would have been to suggest reducing intake of carbohydrates and fat *and* cholesterol. But if you've ever tried to do this, you know that you can eliminate fats *or* carbs, but cutting out both is difficult. You simply run out of things to eat.

In addition to a growing awareness of the seriousness of obesity and diabetes, it had begun to dawn on me—as it had on many cardiologists—that the standard low-fat, low-cholesterol diet we had recommended for years did not prevent heart disease. On the other hand, new cholesterol-lowering medications, called *statins*, were yielding astonishing results. One pill a day could reduce cholesterol levels by 30 to 50 percent and drop the risk of heart disease by as much as 67 percent.

THEN CAME SYNDROME X

By the early 1990s, it had become apparent that although high blood cholesterol explained why some people developed heart and blood vessel disease, it didn't tell the whole story. Many individuals with normal cholesterol levels developed blocked arteries. In search of more answers, researchers began focusing on something that practicing doctors had noticed for years. Certain laboratory and physical findings tended to occur together in the same individual to raise the risk of heart disease *even when cholesterol levels were normal*. These included the following characteristics:

▶ "Visceral" obesity—a tendency to accumulate fat within the abdomen (commonly called potbelly)

▶ A high blood level of a type of fat called triglyceride

▸ A low blood level of HDL ("good cholesterol")

▸ Borderline high blood-sugar level

▸ A family history of diabetes

▸ Mild high blood pressure

Doctors noticed that these traits often clustered not just in the same individual, but also in certain families. Because researchers didn't know what caused this tendency, they named it Syndrome *X*.

Looking at What Causes Syndrome *X*

It was exciting news when researchers discovered that the cause of Syndrome *X* is insulin resistance. This revelation turned previous notions about nutrition upside down. (See chapters 5 and 6 for more on insulin resistance.)

Insulin resistance is a disorder of *carbohydrate* metabolism that has little to do with fat and cholesterol consumption. Not only does insulin resistance predispose people to heart and blood vessel disease, but it encourages weight gain, brings on diabetes and underlies a host of other medical problems.

Atkins Meets Syndrome *X*

It was curious to me that professional organizations, such as the American Heart Association, didn't change their dietary recommendations in response to the discovery of insulin resistance. Instead, they continued to recommend low-fat, *high*-carbohydrate diets even though these clearly exacerbated the condition. The thinking was that even though people with insulin resistance tolerated carbohydrates poorly, it was inappropriate to warn them against eating such foods, because it might encourage them to eat more fat and cholesterol, which was anathema at the time.

In the early 1990s, Dr. Atkins published an updated version of his book, *Dr. Atkins' New Diet Revolution*, and people started trying his low-carbohydrate approach again. Predictably, I started seeing patients with Syndrome *X* who had been on the Atkins Diet. I had laboratory results on many of these individuals going back for years, so I was able to observe any change. I saw astonishing results: waistlines shrinking, triglyceride levels plummeting, and good cholesterol concentrations rising. Remarkably, despite a higher intake of fat- and cholesterol-containing foods, bad cholesterol levels didn't rise much. In fact, they usually went down!

I remember one of my Syndrome *X* patients who made a special appointment to see me because he thought he had cancer. He had gone on the Atkins Diet to lose weight, and, despite generous amounts of rich food, he was dropping pounds so fast it frightened him. I was glad to inform him that he didn't have cancer, and he hadn't been this healthy in years.

Then, as now, it was obvious that for patients with insulin resistance, an Atkins-type diet was the best way to go. It didn't matter if they ate meat and dairy products. If they avoided starchy foods, they lost weight, felt great, and their blood tests looked better. I was convinced—and still am—that for people with Syndrome *X*, a low-carb diet, with plenty of red meat, eggs, and dairy products, is superior to the standard low-cholesterol, high-carbohydrate regimen. Indeed, recent research study results published in the United States' most prestigious medical journal, the *New England Journal of Medicine* (May 22, 2003), have confirmed that low-carbohydrate diets are better than low-fat diets for losing weight, lowering triglycerides, raising HDL, and relieving insulin resistance, and that bad cholesterol levels rarely rise significantly. In fact, they usually go down.

What about People with High Cholesterol?

As helpful as the Atkins approach was for people with Syndrome *X*, I soon encountered a dilemma. Many of my Syndrome *X* patients who would have benefited from a low-carbohydrate diet also had high blood cholesterol. At first, I was hesitant to recommend the Atkins approach to them, because I was afraid it would raise their cholesterol levels. Then, in the late 1990s, doctors who treated patients with high blood cholesterol began noticing something interesting. Patients who took cholesterol-lowering medication were often better off eating *more* fat and cholesterol and reducing their starch and sugar intake. As with Syndrome *X* patients, their triglycerides fell, their good cholesterol levels rose, and their bad cholesterol levels either didn't change much or went down. In effect, the medication took care of the cholesterol side of their body chemistry, and the low-carb diet took care of the carbohydrate side.

In one study, each individual in a group of heart patients on cholesterol medication ate a pound and a half of meat and cheese a day but restricted starch intake. In six weeks, the study subjects lost an average of ten pounds of body fat, their cholesterol levels dropped, and their carbohydrate metabolism improved dramatically.

I don't suggest that you eat more fat than you're naturally inclined to. However, I now routinely recommend low-starch, liberalized-fat diets to Syndrome *X* patients who have high blood cholesterol, once their levels have been lowered with medication.

THE (UNMODIFIED) ATKINS DIET IS NOT FOR EVERYBODY

If you have Syndrome X or diabetes, you are better off focusing your efforts on reducing starch and sugar than worrying about the cholesterol in your diet. But here's the bad news. The increased intake of saturated fat and cholesterol of an unmodified Atkins Diet pushes some people's levels up too high. This is most likely to occur if you have a genetic flaw in your cholesterol-removing mechanisms. Although a low-carb diet may still be your best strategy, you may need to modify your fat and cholesterol intake or take cholesterol-lowering medication. In other words, you need to tailor your diet and medications to your particular body chemistry (see part 3).

There is no one-size-fits-all diet to lower cholesterol, alleviate insulin resistance, and lose weight. You have to match your diet, exercise patterns, and medication to your particular metabolic type. To know what kind of program is right for you, you need to assess your body's ability to handle dietary carbohydrates and cholesterol. That can be easily accomplished by looking at the results of some basic blood tests—which you have probably already had—and the answers to a few questions about your medical history. Later I will show you exactly how to do it (chapters 6–8).

KEY IDEAS FOR TAKEOUT

- Syndrome X is the tendency for the following conditions to occur together in the same individual: fat accumulation in the abdomen, high blood triglyceride level, low good cholesterol (HDL) level, mild high blood-pressure, and a borderline high blood-glucose level or a family history of diabetes.

- Syndrome X is caused by insulin resistance, a disorder of carbohydrate metabolism that has nothing to do with dietary cholesterol.

- Insulin resistance raises the risk of heart disease even if blood cholesterol levels are normal.

- Most overweight people have insulin resistance.

- The best treatment for insulin resistance is a low-carb, liberalized-fat diet combined with moderate exercise.

- Low-carbohydrate diets encourage fat consumption whereas low-fat diets encourage carbohydrate consumption.

- The increased saturated-fat consumption that typically accompanies low-carb diets sometimes raises blood cholesterol, espeically if you have a genetic flaw in your cholesterol metabolism.

- Low-carb, liberalized-fat diets are okay for people with high blood cholesterol if their cholesterol level is controlled with medication.

CHAPTER 3

Cholesterol Demystified

Losing weight requires making some lifestyle changes, and you can't afford to waste your resources on things that won't help you lose weight—and that includes misdirected efforts to fight cholesterol.

But, weight fluctuations that result when you try to lower your cholesterol can confuse the issue. You have to remember that removing any concentrated source of calories from the diet encourages weight loss, and, as weight falls, cholesterol levels usually plummet, too. But much of this is caused by a fall in triglycerides. Once weight stabilizes at a lower level, your bad cholesterol level usually drifts back up. In other words, this means that although you may lose weight and watch your bad cholesterol level decrease initially, the situation won't stay that way in the long run.

MIXED MESSAGING

Let me give you an example of a patient of mine who was sidetracked from a realistic weight-loss program by her cholesterol concerns.

> **W**hen Jean graduated from high school, she weighed 110 pounds, but in her thirties and forties, she gained 40 pounds—mainly around her abdomen. When Jean was fifty-three, her doctor diagnosed a borderline high blood-glucose level, high blood pressure, and a high triglyceride level. In hopes of losing weight and lowering her cholesterol, Jean became a vegetarian, but when she stopped eating meat, she ate more bread, potatoes, rice, and baked goods. In the next two years, she gained 30 more pounds and developed type 2 diabetes.

Jean had all the attributes of Syndrome X (see chapter 2) and insulin resistance (see chapters 5 and 6). She didn't need a low-cholesterol diet. A low-starch diet would have been more appropriate, but when she became a vegetarian, she started eating more starch and sugar, which aggravated her tendency to gain weight and brought on diabetes.

Make no mistake, cholesterol is important. Infiltration of blood vessels by this substance is the number-one cause of heart attacks. Nothing—not surgery, blood thinners, or any other kind of medication—prevents heart attacks better than lowering blood concentrations of cholesterol. For the sake of your health, you have to make the right decision when it comes to cholesterol. On the other hand, you can't let cholesterol concerns distract you from your goal of losing weight. That means your cholesterol strategy has to be exactly right, too, just as your weight-loss strategy.

UNDERSTANDING HOW YOUR BODY PROCESSES CHOLESTEROL

So, what is this substance that everybody worries so much about? And what can you do to keep it out of your arteries?

To understand how your body handles cholesterol and carbohydrates, you need to know about the three kinds of cholesterol particles in your bloodstream: triglycerides, LDL (bad cholesterol), and HDL (good cholesterol).

Contrary to common belief, most of the cholesterol in your bloodstream doesn't come from meat and dairy products. Your liver makes it, about three times as much as you eat. In fact, if you eat less, it just manufactures more. It's a vital component of cells, hormones, and other important things.

In addition to cholesterol, which has the consistency of toothpaste, your liver also makes fat—a vital component of cells and hormones and a major source of energy for muscles. The fat your liver makes is called triglyceride, which has the consistency of olive oil.

Triglycerides

Before your liver can send triglyceride and cholesterol through the bloodstream to tissues that need them, it has to find a way to transport them in the bloodstream, and this presents two problems. First, triglyceride and cholesterol are oil, blood is mainly water, and oil and water don't mix. Recall what happens when you stop shaking a bottle of oil-and-vinegar salad dressing. The oil comes out of solution. The second problem is that cholesterol is damaging to arteries. It can seep into the crevices in arteries, build up there, and cause damage.

The liver handles these problems by bundling cholesterol and triglyceride together into tiny packets and coating them with a layer of emulsifying agent to hold them in solution. This not only solves the oil-and-water dilemma, it also keeps cholesterol from damaging arteries. Although the packets are too small for even a microscope to see, they're too big to get into crevices. They float harmlessly through the bloodstream, held in solution by their coat of emulsifying agent.

As those packets leave your liver, they are called *very-low-density lipoprotein*. Think of them as "floaters." They drift through your bloodstream without settling into your arteries.

Doctors don't usually measure floaters directly. It's much easier to measure triglyceride, which reflects the number of floaters. When your doctor talks about your triglyceride level, he is referring to the number of floaters in your blood.

Here's why your blood-triglyceride level is important:

▶ An excess concentration of triglyceride reduces the levels of HDL or "good cholesterol" in your blood, which promotes atherosclerosis even if your bad cholesterol level is normal.

▶ A high triglyceride concentration is a reliable indicator of insulin resistance. When you consume more carbohydrate than your body can efficiently handle, your liver converts it to triglyceride. The opposite is also true. If you have Syndrome *X* (see chapter 2) and you exercise and restrict starch and sugar, dependably, within days, your blood triglyceride level will plummet.

Bad Cholesterol

As floaters pass through your circulation, the parts of your body that need triglyceride help themselves, leaving most of the cholesterol behind. As a result, the packets get smaller, heavier, and richer in cholesterol. After they have lost most of their triglyceride, they are referred to as *low-density lipoprotein* (LDL) or "bad cholesterol" or "sinkers." In contrast to floaters, sinkers are small enough to settle into crevices in arteries, lodge there, and cause damage.

We all have LDL sinkers in our bloodstream, and as long as the levels aren't too high, our bodies can keep up with the job of cleaning them out. But too many sinkers can overwhelm the mechanisms for removing them and cause cholesterol to accumulate in the walls of our arteries, and this *infiltration by LDL packets is, in fact, what causes atherosclerosis.*

Your first line of defense against a high blood-LDL level is your liver. Tiny receptors on the surface of liver cells pluck LDL packets out of your bloodstream. But some people's LDL receptors don't work very well; the liver can't remove LDL packets efficiently enough, so they back up in the bloodstream. *Inefficient removal of LDL packets—not excessive dietary intake of fat or cholesterol—causes the high-blood cholesterol levels that lead to artery disease.*

Good Cholesterol

The third type of cholesterol particle in your blood is high-density lipoprotein (HDL) or "good cholesterol." HDL packets work like vacuum cleaners that circulate through your body sucking up loose cholesterol that has been deposited by LDL in the walls of arteries. In contrast to LDL, which clogs your blood vessels, HDL helps keep your arteries clean.

A high HDL level helps protect your blood vessels from cholesterol buildup. The more HDL you have in your blood, the less likely you are to develop atherosclerosis. For example, a one-point increase in your good cholesterol lowers your risk as much as a three-point decrease in your bad cholesterol level. If you have a high cholesterol level that is the result of high HDL concentrations, your chances of developing artery disease may actually be lower than average. On the other hand, if you have a low cholesterol level, you may still be at risk if total HDL is low. That's one reason you should not rely on your blood cholesterol levels alone to guide your treatment. You need to take into consideration the levels of all three kinds of cholesterol particles.

Although excess triglycerides in the blood lower good cholesterol, your HDL level is largely genetically determined. Although some medications raise good cholesterol levels, the best treatment currently for a low HDL level is to maintain a low LDL level.

Seeing Signposts for Treatment

You can see that the three kinds of cholesterol packets in your blood are indicators of what's going on in the cholesterol and carbohydrate sides of your metabolism. Although LDL is what gets into your arteries, your triglyceride and HDL levels are also important pieces of information that can help guide you toward the right strategy—not only for lowering your cholesterol, but also for losing weight and preventing diabetes.

Here are the important facts:

▸ A high LDL level indicates your liver is having trouble removing cholesterol packets from your bloodstream.

▸ A high triglyceride concentration or low HDL level suggests that your body is having trouble handling carbohydrates.

FIGURING OUT WHERE YOU STAND

Doctors estimate LDL by measuring the total blood cholesterol concentration and subtracting the cholesterol contained in packets other than LDL—that is, in floaters and HDL, good cholesterol. Here's the formula: total cholesterol *minus* HDL *minus* one-fifth of the triglyceride. If you're unsure of your math, call your doctor's office and ask the staff what your last LDL level was. It's usually right on the laboratory report. Also, ask for your HDL and triglyceride levels while you're at it.

Once you know your LDL level, the next step is to figure out if it's high enough to pose a risk. It is important to understand that there is no sharp cutoff between normal and abnormal. The chances that a particular blood level of LDL will cause trouble depend on the presence of other risk factors. These include a low blood-HDL level, cigarette smoking, diabetes, high blood pressure, and/or a family history of heart disease. If you have one or more of those risk factors, an LDL level that would otherwise be safe may mean trouble. On the other hand, a high blood level of good cholesterol lowers the risk; in other words, if your HDL is high, an LDL that might otherwise be too high may be okay.

Doing the Math

The National Cholesterol Education Program (NCEP), a division of the National Institutes of Health, has developed a simple but effective method to help doctors decide when to recommend cholesterol-lowering treatment. It's considered the gold standard by most heart specialists, and I strongly recommend that you probably follow its recommendations.

Here's how to tell if your LDL level is too high:

▸ If it is less than 130, unless you have signs of atherosclerosis or diabetes, you probably don't need to lower it further.

▸ If it's higher than 130, answer the questions in Table 3.1, and score like this: Give yourself one point for every "yes" answer, zero for every "no" answer; then add up the points.

Table 3.1		
Are you a male over 45 or a female over 55 years?	+	
Smoke cigarettes?	+	
Have high blood pressure (treated or untreated)?	+	
A family history of *early* heart disease (an immediate family member, below age 65)?	+	
Low HDL (male below 40, female below 50)?	+	
High HDL (above 60)? *Subtract one point*	-	
TOTAL POINTS	=	

If your score is zero or one, an LDL level lower than 160 is okay. If your score is two or more, your level should be less than 130, with the following two exceptions:

1. If you already have a narrow or blocked artery or if you have type 2 diabetes, the risk of future artery problems is high enough that the guidelines recommend you get your LDL level below 100, whether you have other risk factors or not. For most people, that requires cholesterol-lowering medication.

2. If you have already evidence of artery disease, many doctors are now recommending that you try to get your LDL level below 75. That's lower than the American Heart Association guidelines recommends, but there's evidence that aiming for 75 is more likely to reverse cholesterol buildup than using 100 as a target.

Knowing What to Do Next

Once you know the levels of the three kinds of cholesterol in your blood, you and your doctor can consult the guidelines and decide if you need to lower your LDL level. The guidelines also indicate how low it should be. The next question is how to get your LDL level where it needs to be and keep it there.

KEY IDEAS FOR TAKEOUT

- You have three kinds of cholesterol particles in your blood: bad cholesterol, good cholesterol, and triglycerides.

- Inefficient removal—not excessive dietary intake—causes high blood levels of bad cholesterol.

- Low-fat, low-cholesterol diets are usually inadequate for treating high blood cholesterol, and because they often rely on increased dietary carbohydrates, they may worsen insulin resistance or diabetes.

- High triglyceride levels usually mean insulin resistance.

- Excess triglycerides wash away good cholesterol.

- This chapter contains guidelines issued by the NCEP for deciding if you should take measures to reduce blood levels of bad cholesterol.

CHAPTER 4

High Blood Cholesterol: Lifestyle or Genes?

For the most part, it's not your diet that determines whether you have a high blood-cholesterol level. It's your genetic makeup. Common hereditary defects in the body's mechanisms for removing cholesterol from the bloodstream are hardwired into some people's genes—they inherit them. You can modify the effects of those flaws with diet and exercise, but you can't change the blueprint.

FACING THE REALITY OF GENETICS

Look at it this way: a month of eating steak and eggs might drive your cholesterol up 5 or 10 percent, but a genetic quirk can triple it.

Consider the experiences of two patients of mine:

> **V**icki has a severe defect of cholesterol metabolism. Half of her blood relatives have been affected. Her son died of a heart attack when he was thirty-one. Her nephew developed severe coronary artery disease at the age of twenty-eight. Although she had been on a strict low-cholesterol diet for years, by the time she was fifty-five, she had coronary artery disease and narrowing of the vessels leading to her brain, intestines, and legs. She seemed destined to die within a few years.

No amount of willpower and discipline could have corrected the hereditary defects that caused Vicki's high cholesterol. Happily, though, she actually has lived into her late eighties, but not because she ate bean sprouts and exercised. She sought medical advice and got on medication that lowered her cholesterol level. This reversed her artery disease and gave her a long and healthy life.

For every patient like Vicki, however, there are several more like Peter.

Peter is a busy executive who has let himself go. At the age of fifty-two, he's obese, lives on junk food, and doesn't exercise. He feels unhealthy and is frustrated by his weight. However, his blood-cholesterol level is lower than 90 percent of the population's.

It seems unfair, doesn't it? Although Peter may still run into problems related to his obesity and sedentary lifestyle, he was lucky enough to be the heir to a good set of cholesterol-metabolizing genes.

LACK OF WILLPOWER ISN'T THE PROBLEM

Don't beat yourself up over your cholesterol count. Lack of discipline didn't raise your cholesterol—your genes did. You may wish you had more strength of character that would help you "fix" your high-cholesterol problem, but you don't need a personal epiphany to lower your cholesterol count. Besides, keeping your arteries healthy is too important to entrust to human willpower.

If your cholesterol level is genuinely high, you need a bombproof way to get it down, and there are easier, more effective ways to get the job done than depriving yourself of good food.

Weighing the Myths and Realities of High Cholesterol

We've all been bombarded by images of people exercising relentlessly and eating vegetables, suggesting they were beating back artery disease with sheer willpower and determination. But lowering cholesterol isn't about some test of inner strength. The notion that your blood cholesterol level is a direct reflection of your lifestyle is misleading.

Here are the facts:

▶ **You can't eat your way to a low cholesterol level.** Diet isn't much help for lowering cholesterol. Strictly supervised low-fat, low-cholesterol diets reduce blood levels of bad cholesterol on average from 5 to 10 percent. If you compare that to the effects of modern cholesterol-lowering medications, which can lower those levels by 50 percent, you can see that low-cholesterol diets start looking like a lot of deprivation for little gain. In fact, most carefully controlled research studies show such diets have little effect on heart attack and death rates.

▶ **You can't exercise high cholesterol away.** Exercise improves endurance and well-being whether you have heart disease or not, and it's the most effective way to lose weight, alleviate insulin resistance, and prevent diabetes. Exercise also raises your blood level of HDL (good cholesterol). But, in spite of these benefits, research shows that even vigorous exercise has little effect on your blood level of LDL (bad cholesterol)—the stuff that actually gets in your arteries and causes atherosclerosis.

▶ **Stopping smoking won't lower your cholesterol.** Giving up smoking is the single most important lifestyle change you can make to reduce your risk of heart disease, cancer, and emphysema. Smoking directly damages arteries and triggers blood clots, which are especially devastating (see part 5).

If you quit smoking, the odds of heart attack begin to decline within days. After two years, they're no higher than if you had never smoked.

However, as harmful as smoking is, it doesn't actually raise cholesterol levels. Giving up the habit won't lower them.

▸ **Don't believe the "good old days" myth.** People are fond of saying that Americans wouldn't have clogged arteries if they lived a more natural lifestyle. What's needed, the argument goes, is a return to the "old" ways—eating like homesteaders and leading less stressful lives. People in this mindset often distrust medical treatment because it is unnatural.

What they tend to overlook is the dramatic change in life expectancy. Until the twentieth century, the average life span was less than fifty years. People didn't live long enough to worry about atherosclerosis. The reason that heart disease is so much more common today has nothing to do with junk food or stress. It's because—thanks to better nutrition, control of infectious diseases, and good obstetrical care— we're living long enough to get atherosclerosis.

▸ **Medication can finesse genetics.** For years, strict low-fat, low-cholesterol diets—though marginally effective—were the only treatment available for high blood cholesterol. But there are more effective options now. Scientists have solved the mystery of what goes wrong with the body's metabolic machinery to cause high blood cholesterol. Now, safe, easy-to-take medications can open the genetic logjam that causes high blood cholesterol.

CORRECTING THE DYSFUNCTION

By correcting the metabolic quirk that leads to high blood levels of LDL, you can prevent and even reverse atherosclerosis. In fact, if you really do have high blood cholesterol that you can't easily control with lifestyle changes and you're not taking one of these medications to lower it, you're missing out on one of the most valuable advances in the history of medicine. See your doctor and find out if one of these medications can get you on the road to lowering your cholesterol, and concentrate on controlling your weight with lifestyle changes.

KEY IDEAS FOR TAKEOUT

- Your cholesterol level is largely genetically determined.

- Lifestyle changes are only marginally helpful for lowering bad cholesterol levels.

- Modern cholesterol medications successfully neutralize the genetic defect that causes high cholesterol.

- Strictly supervised low-cholesterol diets reduce blood levels of bad cholesterol by between 5 and 10 percent on average. Modern cholesterol-lowering medications can reduce them by 50 percent.

CHAPTER 5

The Scourge of the New Millennium: Obesity and its Henchman, Diabetes

ndustrial nations of the world are in the midst of an epidemic of obesity, and the United States is leading the charge. About 64 percent of us are overweight by at least fifteen pounds, and thirty percent are grossly obese, defined as more than fifty pounds overweight, lugging around so much weight we're physically handicapped.

What's frightening is that these numbers are climbing rapidly and show no signs of slowing down. Obesity rates are rising especially fast among the young.

BEING FAT ISN'T JOLLY

This is a sad situation. Fatness is not only unhealthy, it's also psychologically debilitating. It strikes at the core of a person's self-esteem. Obesity adversely affects people's relationships, their ability to participate in activities, and their potential for employment. Indeed, an alarming number of people in the United States can't work for the simple reason that they are too fat.

This epidemic has taken the medical profession by surprise. Most doctors have been trained to deal with what were considered "real diseases," and being overweight has long been regarded as a cosmetic issue. However, doctors are finally starting to treat obesity as the serious health threat it is.

For most people, the desire to avoid obesity has more to do with the fact that our society considers it unattractive than with the health consequences. However, being fat is not just about appearance; it causes a host of medical problems, including high blood pressure, varicose veins, blood clots, gallbladder disease, hip and knee arthritis, and back trouble. Obesity even raises the risk of certain kinds of cancer. The most common, direct, and troublesome complication of obesity, however, is diabetes.

DIABETES IS REACHING EPIDEMIC PROPORTIONS

Diabetes is an inability of the body to remove glucose, a breakdown product of starch and sugar, from the bloodstream. The two kinds are type 1 and type 2.

Looking at Type 1

Type 1, also called *juvenile diabetes*, usually comes on in childhood or early adulthood and is caused by a deficiency of *insulin*, a hormone that allows glucose to pass out of the bloodstream into various bodily tissues. This type of diabetes results from damage to the insulin-secreting cells of the pancreas, a gland about the size of your hand that lies behind your stomach. It is triggered by a viral infection and has little to do with lifestyle.

Understanding Type 2

Type 2 diabetes, sometimes called adult-onset diabetes, usually comes on in midlife. It is much more common than type 1. About 10 percent of adults older than fifty have it, and the percentages are rising rapidly. In contrast to those with type 1, individuals with type 2 usually make adequate amounts of insulin, but their bodies don't respond to it normally. This kind of diabetes has everything to do with lifestyle. Excessive body fat and sedentary living bring it on by reducing the body's sensitivity to insulin. Successful treatment requires close attention to diet and exercise.

The incidence of type 2 diabetes has skyrocketed along with the obesity rate. As a practical matter, if you're an American older than forty, you're much more likely to develop type 2 diabetes than heart disease in the next ten years.

High glucose levels in the blood caused by both types of diabetes can literally sugarcoat bodily tissues. After several years, poorly controlled diabetes may damage eyes, kidneys, and nerves. Diabetes is the number-one cause of blindness, kidney failure, and lower-limb amputations in the United States. But the main source of trouble is artery disease.

Although type 2 diabetes doesn't raise bad cholesterol levels, it leads to artery damage in other ways. High concentrations of glucose in the blood damage arteries directly. In addition, the insulin resistance that usually accompanies type 2 diabetes reduces levels of protective substances in the blood and alters bad cholesterol in ways that makes it especially harmful to arteries.

On the Way to Trouble without Knowing It

In the past, you were classified as having diabetes only if your body showed marked difficulty in handling carbohydrates; that is, if you couldn't maintain normal blood levels of glucose. However, doctors now know that many people have mild forms of diabetes, and many with borderline high levels of blood sugar or transient elevations go on to develop the disease. These prediabetics are often unaware of their susceptibility, and in blissful ignorance of their health status, they consume a diet high in refined carbohydrates, which exacerbates mild diabetes and quickens the progression to more flagrant disease.

SPOTTING THE TROUBLEMAKER

Insulin resistance is the term doctors use to describe a disorder of carbohydrate metabolism—in which people's bodies lose sensitivity to their own insulin. (See more on insulin resistance in chapter 6.)

Poor eating habits and sedentary living aggravate insulin resistance and promote weight gain. Excess body fat, in turn, leads to more insulin resistance. The spiral of increasing weight and worsening insulin resistance sets the stage for type 2 diabetes.

Insulin resistance can cause artery disease even without

diabetes, but it's especially likely to cause trouble if it has progressed to diabetes. The two routes to heart and blood vessel disease: (1) through genetic defects of the body's mechanisms for removing cholesterol and (2) through obesity, insulin resistance, and diabetes.

KEY IDEAS FOR TAKEOUT

- America is experiencing an epidemic of obesity, which has led to a skyrocketing incidence of type 2 diabetes.

- Obesity unmasks insulin resistance, which, in turn, worsens obesity and leads to type 2 diabetes.

- Insulin resistance leads to heart disease even when diabetes is absent.

- There are two routes to heart disease, via high blood cholesterol and via insulin resistance.

PART 2
SETTING UP A PROGRAM THAT WORKS FOR YOU

You've never lost weight and kept it off? You recognize the fallacies in one-diet-for-all-people? You're looking for a way to become healthier but have struck out so far?

Part 2 of *The New Low-Carb Way* will help you design a program specifically for your body chemistry. It will show you how to profile your body chemistry and design a strategy for your particular metabolic type.

You will discover the easiest, most efficient way to lose weight, prevent diabetes, and keep your heart healthy in the bargain.

CHAPTER 6

Insulin Resistance: How Does Your Body Handle Carbohydrates?

If you have gained more than thirty pounds since high school, there's a good chance that you have insulin resistance, the most common metabolic disturbance known. Overall, insulin resistance affects about 22 percent of adult Americans—44 percent of those older than fifty. It's especially common among adults with excessive midlife weight gain.

But even though insulin resistance is common, it's certainly not harmless. This is the number-one known cause of obesity. Insulin resistance also predisposes an individual to heart disease, diabetes, and a host of other serious medical conditions.

What is insulin resistance, how can you tell if you have it, and how do you get rid of it?

UNDERSTANDING INSULIN RESISTANCE

If you are insulin resistant, your body makes plenty of insulin but doesn't respond to it normally. To allow glucose to pass out of your bloodstream and into your body's tissues, your pancreas has to secrete as much as six times the normal amount of insulin. Excessive insulin makes you gain weight, raises your triglyceride levels, and lowers your HDL, which predisposes you to artery disease.

Many people are genetically predisposed to insulin resistance. However, it doesn't manifest itself until lifestyle factors bring it out. Sedentary living and excessive consumption of refined carbohydrates unmask the genetic tendency. In addition, obesity itself worsens insulin resistance. It's a classic vicious cycle: Weight gain aggravates insulin resistance; insulin resistance promotes weight gain.

Because insulin resistance is mainly a disorder of muscle metabolism—and the other cells of the body remain largely unaffected—you can decrease or increase your muscles' responsiveness to insulin by how you use them. (In chapter 15, you will learn how you can alleviate insulin resistance by activating your muscle metabolism.)

DIAGNOSING INSULIN RESISTANCE

You might think that diagnosing insulin resistance is easy—just measure blood-insulin levels. The problem is, insulin disappears so quickly from the bloodstream that it's difficult to measure. To find out if you're insulin resistant, you start with a diabetes check.

Diagnosing diabetes is straightforward. You have your blood-glucose level checked; if you find out that it's high, you will know that you probably have diabetes, and if it's normal, you probably don't. The American Diabetes Association defines "normal" as a fasting blood-glucose concentration less than 126.

Some doctors are hesitant to label patients with mild elevations of blood glucose—in the range of 126 to 140—as having diabetes. Make no mistake, if you haven't eaten for twelve hours and your blood sugar is 126 or higher, your body isn't handling carbohydrates normally. (If your doctor isn't concerned, find one who is.)

If your fasting blood-glucose level is in the high-normal range—from 110 to 125—you don't have true diabetes, but you are at increased risk of developing it. Also, if your blood-glucose level rises more than usual after a starchy meal—higher than 180—you have what's called glucose intolerance, which often progresses to type 2 diabetes.

LOOKING FOR SIGNS OF INSULIN RESISTANCE

If your answer is yes to any three of the following five

questions, you probably have insulin resistance.

1. Do you tend to accumulate fat within your abdomen?

If you're a man and your waist measurement is larger than forty inches, or if you're a woman and it's larger than thirty-five inches, you probably have insulin resistance. However, even if your waist measurement doesn't exceed that limit, a tendency to concentrate fat in your abdomen as opposed to elsewhere on your body is strongly suggestive of insulin resistance. If your belly protrudes, even if you're not flabby elsewhere, that's a sign that you're insulin resistant.

An accurate way to determine if you accumulate fat in your abdomen is to calculate your waist-to-hip ratio. Measure your girth around your navel and your hip circumference around your buttocks, and divide your waist measurement by your hip reading. A waist circumference larger than 95 percent of your hip girth if you're a male, or 85 percent of your hip circumference if you're a female, is a reliable sign of insulin resistance, even if you are not markedly overweight.

2. Is your blood triglyceride level high?

A high blood level of triglyceride signals insulin resistance. If you're insulin resistant, your body will have trouble handling the glucose released in your bloodstream by carbohydrates, so your liver will convert it to triglyceride. Healthy people without insulin resistance usually have triglyceride levels less than 125. A level greater than 150 suggests insulin resistance. If it's more than 200, you almost certainly have insulin resistance.

3. Is your "good cholesterol" level low?

Take into consideration the fact that women naturally have higher HDL levels than men do. An HDL level below 40 for a man or 50 for a woman is a sign of insulin resistance.

A low HDL often reflects *previously* high triglyceride levels. Triglyceride changes rapidly. A few days of carbohydrate restriction or exercise can lower your levels substantially. If you have been avoiding starch and sugar and exercising for a few days preceding your blood test, it might miss a previously high level. However, HDL provides a clue. Low HDL levels caused by high triglyceride stay low for several days after the triglyceride levels go back down. A blood test that misses a high triglyceride may detect a low HDL.

4. Is your blood pressure mildly elevated?

Even mildly elevated blood pressure readings increase the likelihood that you have insulin resistance. The pressure of the blood in your arteries rises and falls with each beat of your heart. The high point is called the *systolic* pressure, and the low point, the *diastolic* pressure. Normally, the systolic pressure is 130 or less, and the diastolic below 85. In the past, doctors diagnosed high blood pressure if the systolic pressure exceeded 145 or the diastolic, 95. However, many people with insulin resistance have blood pressures in the borderline range—systolic pressures between 130 and 145, diastolic pressures between 85 and 95.

5. Do you have borderline high blood-glucose levels or a family history of type 2 diabetes?

Doctors often ignore blood-glucose readings between 110 and 126. However, fasting glucose levels in that range suggest insulin resistance and raise the likelihood of future type 2 diabetes. Also, immediate family members of people with type 2 diabetes often have insulin resistance. If one of your parents or a sibling has type 2 diabetes, there's a good chance you have insulin resistance. (That is not true for type 1 diabetes, which is less hereditable.)

The Sugar in Your Coffee Is Different from the "Sugar" in Your Blood

Misunderstanding the meaning of the word *sugar* often results in misdirected dietary efforts to treat insulin resistance and diabetes. Although the building block of carbohydrate is glucose, doctors and nutritionists have gotten in the habit of saying "sugar." This innocent substitution creates a lot of confusion and can lead to some frustrating problems.

For most people, the word *sugar* means table sugar, the stuff we add to foods to make them sweet. But table sugar is actually sucrose, a double molecule containing one molecule of glucose and one of fructose, making it only half glucose. On the other hand, refined carbohydrates like bread, potatoes, and rice are almost all glucose. Although they're not as sweet to the taste as sucrose, they release about twice the amount of glucose into your bloodstream.

UNCHECKED INSULIN RESISTANCE CAN HAVE MAJOR CONSEQUENCES

Insulin is a powerful hormone. An overdose of insulin medication can kill a person. It has even been used as a murder weapon. Thus, it's not surprising that excessive secretion, over years, can create serious medical problems. Here are some of the consequences:

Type 2 diabetes. After years of excessive insulin production, the pancreas often seems to burn out. Insulin secretion can no longer keep up with demand, and blood-glucose levels finally rise. The result is type 2 diabetes.

Whether a person with insulin resistance goes on to develop type 2 diabetes depends on how severe the insulin resistance is and how well the pancreas holds up under the strain. Some people's pancreases burn out faster than others'. Even mild insulin resistance can bring on diabetes in such individuals. Other people can have severe insulin resistance for years and never develop diabetes.

Obesity. Excessive insulin encourages the body to store fat. When a person with insulin resistance finally secretes enough insulin to bring down blood glucose after a meal, the level often falls too fast. This stimulates appetite centers in the brain and trigger hunger. Excessive insulin, whether given as a medication or secreted naturally, invariably causes weight gain.

The fat accumulation associated with insulin resistance usually occurs in early adulthood and midlife. The good news is that overweight people with insulin resistance have better luck losing weight than others. Often, they don't have to starve themselves consciously to shed fat. If they reduce their intake of simple carbohydrates, they can often eat satisfying amounts of fat, protein, and complex carbohydrates and still slim down.

Visceral obesity (potbelly). Men with insulin resistance often look slim from behind, but when you look at them in profile, you can see that their bellies protrude. Fat hasn't accumulated on their buttocks, thighs, or arms; it has gone to their abdomens.

The tendency to accumulate weight within the abdomen is less noticeable in women, because their hips and breasts partially obscure their bellies, and they balance their weight farther back over their hips.

There are two theories about the potbelly associated with insulin resistance. One explanation is that high insulin and triglyceride levels cause fat to be stored within the abdomen. The other theory is that the tendency to accumulate fat in the abdomen is inborn, and because fat in that location is directly upstream from the liver, it predisposes a person to insulin resistance.

Regardless, it's a fact that people with insulin resistance tend to have potbellies.

Sleep apnea. Visceral obesity is often accompanied by fat accumulation in the neck. In fact, a thick neck is often a sign of insulin resistance. Fat accumulation in the structures of the neck impinges on air passage through the throat. Consequently, overweight people with insulin resistance often snore heavily during sleep and tend to develop sleep apnea, a condition characterized by erratic breathing that robs sleep of its restfulness. This results in daytime fatigue, drowsiness, and poor concentration. The epidemic of obesity and insulin resistance occurring in developed countries is causing an epidemic of sleep apnea.

High blood triglyceride levels. Most people with insulin resistance have higher-than-normal blood triglyceride levels. Just as cholesterol in the blood doesn't come from cholesterol in the diet, triglyceride, which is, indeed, a fat (see chapter 3), doesn't come from dietary fat. When people eat more carbohydrates than their bodies can handle, their livers convert the excess carbohydrates into the same kind of fat that low-fat diets are designed to avoid.

Low levels of good cholesterol. Excess triglyceride in the blood depletes or "washes away" good cholesterol. People with insulin resistance often have low blood HDL levels, which is the main reason they are susceptible to heart and artery disease.

High blood pressure. Excessive insulin raises blood pressure slightly, which may be why people with insulin resistance usually have blood pressure that is at least mildly elevated. However, other factors are involved in causing high blood pressure, so treatment of insulin resistance alone usually doesn't correct it.

Polycystic ovary syndrome. Gynecologists have noticed for years that women who develop recurrent ovarian cysts tend to have central obesity, menstrual irregularities, and excessive body hair. They call this polycystic ovary syndrome, or PCOS. It is the most common cause of female infertility in the United States. The incidence of PCOS is rising, and it now affects approximately 6 percent of women.

For years, the cause of PCOS was a mystery, but in the early 1990s, doctors made a serendipitous discovery. Women with PCOS who had diabetes often became pregnant when they started taking pills to relieve insulin resistance. It soon became apparent that insulin resistance caused PCOS.

Women with PCOS are often *markedly* insulin resistant, so it is not surprising that this syndrome is a potent risk factor for future heart disease. As many as 25 percent of women with PCOS go on to develop diabetes, and when they do, their risk of heart disease is *seventeen* times higher than average.

When women go to doctors to find out why they have trouble controlling their weight, often the only condition the doctor checks for is low thyroid-hormone level. PCOS is many times more common than thyroid trouble, but unfortunately, nongynecologists frequently overlook it as a cause for weight gain.

Hypoglycemia. Insulin resistance often causes vague and difficult-to-diagnose symptoms. One frequent complaint is what's commonly called hypoglycemia, or low blood sugar. Hypoglycemia causes lightheadedness, shakiness, and a letdown in energy that typically occurs three or four hours after a meal. Eating relieves the symptoms.

Hypoglycemia is, in fact, a misnomer. Blood-glucose levels are rarely low during these episodes. Three or four hours after a starchy meal, when excessive insulin secretion starts bringing blood-glucose levels down, the levels often fall faster than normal. This sudden drop stimulates the hormone *adrenalin*, which keeps the glucose from falling too low. It is the adrenalin, not low blood-glucose levels, that causes the symptoms typical of so-called hypoglycemia.

Diabetic patients who take too much insulin medication often describe compelling cravings for food. Similarly, people with insulin resistance often have quirky appetites and food cravings at odd times. Characteristically, they eat lightly during the day and heavily at night.

CHANGING EXISTING NOTIONS ABOUT DIET

The reason the discovery of insulin resistance created such a maelstrom in the world of nutrition is that the low-cholesterol, low-fat diets that doctors had been recommending relied on replacing meat and dairy products with starchy foods like bread, potatoes, and rice. But for patients with insulin resistance, a diet high in refined carbohydrates—even if it is low in fat and cholesterol—can bring on diabetes, promote weight gain, reduce levels of protective cholesterols in the blood, and actually *raise* blood-cholesterol levels. In other words, for many patients, what doctors had been recommending for years was wrong.

If you add the number of people in the United States who have insulin resistance to the rapidly expanding ranks of those who have diabetes, you can see that a large portion of the population should be paying more attention to their carbohydrate metabolism and worrying less about dietary cholesterol.

KEY IDEAS FOR TAKEOUT

- Insulin allows glucose to pass out of your blood and into your tissues.

- People with insulin resistance make plenty of insulin, but their bodies become resistant to its effects. Consequently, they have to make as much as five times the normal amount of insulin to handle dietary carbohydrates.

- Excessive insulin secretion promotes weight gain and leads to diabetes, heart disease, and several other serious medical problems.

- Insulin resistance is genetically influenced, but lifestyle factors, including excessive starch intake, obesity, and sedentary living, bring it out.

- You are likely to have insulin resistance if you have any three of the following signs:

    1. A large abdomen
    2. A high blood level of triglyceride
    3. A low blood level of HDL (good cholesterol)
    4. A borderline high blood-glucose level or a family history of diabetes
    5. Mild high blood pressure

CHAPTER 7

Profiling Your Body Chemistry

I n diet, customizing works wonders. No single program works for everybody to lower cholesterol, alleviate insulin resistance, and shed pounds. Because the body's ability to handle dietary carbohydrates and cholesterol varies from one individual to another, you have to tailor your diet to your particular metabolic type.

I am going to help you find out what type you are.

LET'S GET PHYSICAL

To determine what your metabolic type is, you need to know the answers to the following questions:

▶ Do you have insulin resistance or diabetes? (See chapter 6.)

▶ Do you have high levels of bad cholesterol? (See chapter 3.)

Armed with that knowledge, you can decide which strategy you need to follow:

▶ A strategy for improving your carbohydrate metabolism and losing weight

▶ A strategy for reducing your blood cholesterol level

▶ A strategy for both of the above

In chapter 8, I give you the programs for these strategies.

Looking at the Two Sides of Your Body Chemistry

You should be starting to see a pattern by now in the way your body handles cholesterol and the way it handles carbohydrates—one you can't control, the other you can. Insulin resistance, obesity, and diabetes are related to the way your body handles carbohydrates, and these health problems have everything to do with your lifestyle. High blood cholesterol results from inborn weaknesses of enzymes that remove cholesterol from your bloodstream, a metabolic quirk that has little to do with your lifestyle.

Not only are good nutrition and exercise your best weapons against insulin resistance, obesity, and diabetes, but they are your only weapons. There are no good medications for insulin resistance or obesity. On the other hand, you can take a pill for high blood cholesterol. The bottom line is that you will get the best return for your efforts by focusing them on relieving insulin resistance and losing weight rather than trying to lower your blood cholesterol level with diet.

Gathering the Information You Need

To profile your body chemistry, gather estimates of the following (you can get the first three from the results of your most recent blood tests):

▶ Good and bad cholesterol levels. (See chapter 3.)

▶ Triglyceride level. (Higher than 150 is unhealthy.)

▶ Blood-glucose level. (Normal is less than 126.)

▶ Blood pressure. (Do you have high blood pressure? Generally speaking, high is anything that goes above 135/85. Normal is 135/85 or less.)

▶ Waist and waist-to-hip measurements. (Do you have a pot-belly? Are you overweight? See measurement guidelines in chapter 6.)

▶ Family health history. (Is there diabetes and/or heart disease in your family?)

Also, based on what you learned in chapters 3 and 6, weigh into the mix your answers to the following questions:

1. Does your body have trouble removing cholesterol from your blood? (See chapter 3.)

2. Does your body have difficulty handling carbohydrates? (If your blood-glucose level is higher than 126, your body isn't processing carbohydrates normally. See chapter 6.)

3. Do you have both problems?

Now that you've accumulated information, you have a body-chemistry profile that will help you decide which strategy you want to follow:

▸ A strategy for improving your carbohydrate metabolism and losing weight

▸ A strategy for reducing your blood cholesterol level

▸ A strategy for lowering blood cholesterol level, improving carbohydrate metabolism, and losing weight

In chapter 8, I give you the programs for each of the above strategies.

ADDRESSING THE CATCH-22 OF BODY CHEMISTRY

It's important to keep the cholesterol and carbohydrate sides of your body chemistry straight. What's good for one part may not be good for the other. The best way to alleviate insulin resistance or treat diabetes may not be the best approach for lowering cholesterol. Sometimes, you have to address the two sides of your metabolism separately. Here is an example of a patient of mine who benefited from this approach:

Jerry's bad cholesterol level was dangerously high, but he also had signs of insulin resistance—a potbelly and a high blood-triglyceride level. At the age of fifty-two, he developed type 2 diabetes. Jerry worked at a job that required extensive travel and entertainment, so it was difficult for him to control what he ate when he was working. To lower his blood cholesterol level, he thought he should reduce his consumption of fat and cholesterol. But it seemed that the food he ate at restaurants and banquets was loaded with starch, which aggravated his diabetes.

He made little progress in controlling his diabetes or his cholesterol problem until he began taking anticholesterol medication. This brought his bad cholesterol level down to safe levels and allowed him to liberalize his intake of fat and cholesterol. Then he focused his dietary efforts on reducing his consumption of starch, and found that he didn't mind cutting out bread, potatoes, and rice if he could have eggs, red meat, and dairy products in moderation. His diabetes became easier to control, and, as a bonus, he lost several inches around his waist.

Jerry had little success with his high blood cholesterol or his diabetes until he addressed each problem individually. By choosing to use medication for his cholesterol imbalance, he was able to alter his eating patterns in ways that benefited his weight and his diabetes.

DECIDING WHAT TO TREAT WITH DIET, WHAT TO TREAT WITH MEDICATIONS

It would be simple if the remedy for high blood cholesterol was the same as that for losing weight and preventing diabetes, but often this isn't so. Although lifestyle changes don't lower blood levels of bad cholesterol very much, medications are effective even if you don't adhere strictly to a low-cholesterol diet. On the other hand, while medications don't help much with losing weight or preventing diabetes, diet and exercise are effective. This leads to decision-making time; chapter 8 helps you choose the strategy that fits your body-chemistry type.

KEY IDEAS FOR TAKEOUT

- How well your body handles dietary carbohydrates and how well it removes bad cholesterol from your blood are two separate parts of your body chemistry.

- If you have insulin resistance, your body has trouble handling dietary carbohydrates.

- If you have high blood levels of bad cholesterol, your body has trouble removing cholesterol from your blood.

- Knowing why your body chemistry is out of kilter will help you put it back in balance.

CHAPTER 8

Choosing the Right Strategy for Your Body-Chemistry Type

Your body's ability to remove cholesterol from your bloodstream and its ability to handle dietary carbohydrates are largely separate aspects of your body chemistry. You may have trouble with one, the other, or both. Genetic weaknesses of enzymes responsible for removing cholesterol cause high blood cholesterol and have little to do with your eating or exercise habits. Inefficient handling of dietary carbohydrates, on the other hand, causes insulin resistance, obesity, and diabetes, and has a lot to do with diet and exercise.

CUSTOMIZING YOUR HEALTH PLAN

There is no single strategy for simultaneously lowering cholesterol, attaining a healthy body weight, and reducing insulin resistance. You need to tailor your eating patterns, exercise habits, and medications to your particular goal(s) and body-chemistry profile (chapter 7). It's all about customizing.

The first strategy—the one you should follow if you want to lose weight and you have trouble metabolizing carbohydrates—is the Carbohydrate Strategy. The second strategy—the one to use if your body has problems breaking down cholesterol—is the Cholesterol Strategy. The plan to follow if your body has trouble breaking down cholesterol *and* metabolizing carbs is the Combined Strategy.

In assessing your body's ability to handle cholesterol and carbohydrates, remember that there are no sharp dividing lines between normal and abnormal. Insulin resistance can be mild, severe, or any degree in between. The same is true for high blood cholesterol. Some people have severely elevated LDL levels, whereas others are borderline and drift back and forth across the upper limits of normal.

The key to success is concentrating your efforts in ways that will do the most good. If you tailor your diet, exercise, and medical strategy to your metabolic profile, you will be amazed how easily you are able to accomplish your goals.

FOLLOWING THE CARBOHYDRATE STRATEGY

If you have insulin resistance or you want to lose weight *and* your bad cholesterol is normal, the Carbohydrate Strategy is the one for you.

Getting Briefed on Food for the Carb Strategy

Remember that the carbohydrate side of your metabolism is exquisitely sensitive to dietary changes and exercise. If you reduce your intake of high-glucose-shock foods (see chapters 10 and 11) and exercise just a little, even if you don't try to cut calories, you're almost sure to see improvements.

Here's what you should do:

▶ **Eliminate refined carbohydrates.** This is straightforward because the offending foods are few in number. Virtually all of the simple carbohydrates come from five sources: grains, potatoes, rice, corn, and sugar. You can follow a liberalized fat-intake diet much like the one seen in the Atkins Diet for weight reduction.

▶ **Take a moderate approach to cutting out starches.** Typically, people who don't try to eliminate starch totally sustain their efforts better than those who take a radical approach. My advice: continue eating bread, potatoes, rice, and corn, but eat less than one-fourth of what you used to consume. (See chapters 10 and 11 for ways to eliminate glucose shocks.) With such a variety of rich foods to choose from, you may think that eliminating four foods—ones that aren't especially exciting—would be easy. But, you can expect to miss simple carbohydrates for a while.

▶ **Familiarize yourself with the glucose-shock ratings of foods you eat regularly** (see chapters 10 and 11). The glucose-shock ratings in this book will help you monitor the amounts of starch that you typically eat in a serving. Remember that fresh fruits and vegetables make but a minor contribution to most people's total glucose-shock loads.

▶ **Purge your thinking of the cholesterol-scare propaganda you've heard for the past three decades.** Forget what you learned about the dangers of dietary fat and cholesterol, and enjoy red meat, eggs, cheese, butter, oils, salad dressings, and shellfish. Eat until you're satisfied. Just get used to eating fewer refined carbohydrates.

▶ **Don't try to restrict calories—at least, at first.** Just cut out refined carbohydrates and eat normally otherwise and see what happens. If you alleviate insulin resistance, you will probably see your belly shrink, your triglyceride level drop, and your bad cholesterol level go down while you continue to eat heartily.

Considering Medications

Drugs called *insulin sensitizers* partially correct insulin resistance, and although doctors mainly use them to treat people with type 2 diabetes, they are starting to use them for insulin resistance without diabetes. However, insulin sensitizers are only partially effective, not nearly as useful for correcting insulin resistance as, for example, cholesterol-lowering drugs are for lowering LDL.

I consider insulin resistance a serious medical problem even when it hasn't progressed to diabetes, and, increasingly, I am prescribing medications for this condition. Researchers have found that one insulin-sensitizing medication—Metformin—improves insulin resistance, encourages weight loss in some people, and forestalls diabetes. Acarbose, a starch blocker, slows the breakdown of starch in the intestinal tract, improves insulin resistance, and prevents blood-vessel disease.

Prescribing medications for insulin resistance opens the door to treating a lot of people, because most overweight adults have insulin resistance. Actually, I think there is a good argument to be made for treating many of these people with medications. Because we have become accustomed to seeing overweight people, we tend not to take excess body weight seriously, when obesity has serious medical consequences beyond just being bothersome.

At the same time, if there ever was a condition for which a natural approach made sense, insulin resistance is it. Excess refined carbohydrates and physical inactivity cause it. Starch restriction and exercise can cure it.

Get Moving

The carbohydrate side of your metabolism is exquisitely sensitive to exercise. If you have the signs of insulin resistance (see list in chapter 6), chances are you'll be amazed by the results of adding exercise. If you combine a low-glucose-shock diet with a moderate increase in your activity level, you will see your triglyceride level plummet and your good cholesterol level rise, and you should steadily lose weight. Few conditions in medicine are as responsive to lifestyle changes as insulin resistance is.

The best way to improve your sensitivity to insulin is to contract the large muscles of your body repetitively for at least twenty minutes every other day (Chapter 15). Such exercise immediately alleviates insulin resistance, an effect

---

The Super *X*

People I call Super *X*'s have flagrant signs of insulin resistance—very high blood-triglyceride levels (higher than 250), markedly protuberant abdomens, and borderline high blood sugar—and they respond exquisitely to carbohydrate restriction and even mild exercise. When they reduce their intake of starch and walk about twenty minutes every other day or so, they lose weight, their triglyceride levels plummet, and their good cholesterol levels rise.

At the same time, Super *X*'s seem immune to the effects of dietary fat. Often, despite a higher cholesterol intake, their bad cholesterol levels improve. It is as if refined carbohydrates are poisons for these individuals. Seeing this makes me appreciate how much we doctors were missing when we didn't listen to what Atkins had to say thirty years ago.

---

that lasts for about forty-eight hours.

The amount of exercise it takes to counteract insulin resistance is less than you might think: just twenty minutes of walking four times a week. In fact, the difference between doing no exercise and walking twenty minutes is greater than the difference between walking and running. (You don't have to run marathons, you just have to get moving. The couch-potato life is unnatural, and your body abhors it.)

DOING THE CHOLESTEROL STRATEGY

If you have a high blood level of bad cholesterol, as defined by the NCEP guidelines in chapter 3, *and* you have no signs of insulin resistance or diabetes, the Cholesterol Strategy is the one for you to follow.

First, Try Reducing Saturated Fat

The first thing you should do is try reducing the amounts of fat and cholesterol you eat and also pay attention to whether you're eating "good fat" or "bad fat" (see chapter 12). This approach resembles the low-fat, low-cholesterol diet that doctors recommended for years but with a liberalized approach toward good fats and a cautious eye toward avoiding excessive starch. (This is important because our ability to handle carbohydrates diminishes as we age; you may not have insulin resistance now, but there's a good chance you could develop it in the future.)

Remember, however, that research studies have shown repeatedly that low-fat, low-cholesterol diets lower blood cholesterol levels by only 5 to 10 percent and are minimally effective at reducing the risk of heart disease. Unlike insulin resistance, hereditary defects in cholesterol metabolism are only modestly responsive to lifestyle changes.

Exercise Doesn't Remove Cholesterol

Unless you have insulin resistance, exercise doesn't do much to lower bad cholesterol or raise good cholesterol. Nevertheless, exercise will enhance your strength, endurance, and vitality. It will also reduce your risk of type 2 diabetes, and if you already have artery disease, it will improve your circulation.

Trying a Different Tack

If a low-saturated-fat, low-cholesterol diet doesn't reduce your LDL to safe levels, you might try cutting carbohydrates.

I have seen several patients who were slim and trim, had no signs of insulin resistance or diabetes, yet their LDL level improved dramatically when they reduced their consumption of refined carbohydrates. If this works for you, you probably have some degree of insulin resistance, and in that case, you should follow the Combined Strategy (described below).

You can also face reality and take medication if you need it (see chapters 18 and 19). Remember, defects in cholesterol removal are difficult to treat with lifestyle changes alone because they are largely genetic. If your lifestyle didn't cause the problem, putting more effort into diet and exercise probably won't help much. If a change of diet doesn't bring your blood LDL level down, it's important for you to accept the fact that you have an inborn error of metabolism, and consider taking advantage of the highly effective medications available to treat it. The good news is that easy-to-take pills (statins) can completely correct the metabolic defect responsible for high levels of bad cholesterol. One tablet a day can lower your LDL to safe levels and markedly reduce your risk of heart and blood-vessel disease.

USING THE COMBINED STRATEGY

If you are overweight or have signs of insulin resistance and but you also have high blood levels of bad cholesterol, you need to follow the Combined Strategy. Insulin resistance and defective cholesterol metabolism are common conditions, so plenty of people have both.

You have to understand that insulin resistance is highly responsive to diet and exercise, but poorly responsive to medication, while high bad cholesterol levels are poorly responsive to diet and exercise but highly responsive to medication. The approach of the Combined Strategy is two-pronged: one directed at the insulin resistance, the other at the cholesterol defect.

TRYING A NEW FOOD APPROACH

At the outset, decrease your consumption of starch and sugar and do moderate exercise, as if you were following the Carbohydrate Strategy. Why cut carbs first? Fat and cholesterol consumption doesn't directly aggravate insulin resistance, but excessive carbohydrates exacerbate cholesterol problems. If you correct the carbohydrate problem, your insulin resistance will improve and your blood level of bad cholesterol may go down even if you don't reduce cholesterol and fat consumption.

Another reason to start by directing treatment toward the carbohydrate defect is that there's no other option for treating this component. Medication will correct the cholesterol defect, but drugs don't work well for insulin resistance. You have to reduce your intake of refined carbohydrates and increase your exercise level.

Walking a Tightrope
Some advocates of low-carb diets skirt the issue of what happens to LDL when you replace carbohydrates with meat and dairy products. Although low-carb, liberal-fat diets reliably improve insulin resistance, they have unpredictable effects on LDL levels. Usually such diets lower it or don't affect it much. However, sometimes they raise LDL. This is especially likely to happen in individuals who

do *not* have insulin resistance. For such folks, the higher dietary fat may counteract the benefits of cutting carbohydrates. Let me illustrate.

> **B**ill is a Super X. When I met him, he had a very high triglyceride level, a large potbelly, high blood pressure, and a family history of type 2 diabetes. He had little success losing weight until he went on the Atkins Diet. He cut out sweets and starches and ate large amounts of fatty foods including bacon, eggs, sausage, cheese, and steaks, yet he was amazed to find that he could eat all he wanted and still lose weight. In a year, he lost thirty-five pounds, and his triglyceride level plummeted. Despite a much higher dietary-fat content than he had ever consumed, his blood-LDL level fell.

> **H**enry was mildly overweight and had a borderline high LDL when he started the Atkins Diet. He lost fifteen pounds but was disappointed to find that the diet raised his blood-LDL level thirty points—high enough to require corrective action.

The point is, LDL levels can go either way on a low-carb, liberal-fat diet. You just have to check them. If your LDL level goes down when you cut refined carbohydrates and exercise, you've just discovered a way to solve your LDL and carbohydrate problems simultaneously.

Knowing the Danger Zone

One word of warning: if you have a high LDL level, your priorities should be different from what they would be if you were just overweight or had insulin resistance. If you don't stick to your diet and exercise regimen and your LDL drifts back up, it's not just a matter of regaining weight. It will raise your risk of heart and blood-vessel disease. Getting your LDL down should be your *top* priority.

Considering the Hard Way and the Easy Way

If cutting refined carbohydrates doesn't bring your LDL down, you have two options: a hard one that doesn't work very well and an easy one that works like a charm. Let's discuss the more difficult, less effective option first.

The hard way. In addition to cutting out refined carbs, you can try reducing your fat and cholesterol consumption, too. To do that, you need to rely on protein, fruits and vegetables in their natural forms, and "good fats" as calorie sources instead of refined carbohydrates and saturated fat. Because that style of eating is reminiscent of traditional eating patterns in some Mediterranean countries, it is called the Mediterranean Diet.

No matter what you call it, the reality is, eliminating both saturated fats and refined carbohydrates markedly restricts your dietary options. You will find it difficult to arrange meals that conform to your requirements yet provide the variety you crave. But if you are intent on avoiding medications and are confident you can stay on such a regimen indefinitely, it might be worth a try.

The easy way. This brings us to the easier, more effective option. Focus your dietary efforts exclusively on the carbohydrate side of your metabolism and let medication handle the cholesterol defect. If you concentrate on reducing your intake of simple carbohydrates and take a statin-type cholesterol-lowering medication to clear up the genetic logjam in your cholesterol metabolism, your carbohydrate metabolism will improve and your LDL level will drop like a rock.

Cholesterol-lowering medications (see chapter 18), such as Mevacor, Pravachol, Zocor, Lescol, Lipitor, and Crestor, have profoundly affected the treatment of high cholesterol. These medications reduce bad cholesterol levels by up to 50 percent and markedly reduce the risk of heart disease. They are all once-a-day pills that doctors have prescribed to millions of patients with few side effects.

When you take cholesterol-lowering medication, you can usually continue to eat eggs, dairy products, and red meat in moderation. In fact, restricting fat and cholesterol may result in your eating more refined carbohydrates and negate some of the beneficial effects of medication.

KEY IDEAS FOR TAKEOUT

- Once you know how well your body handles carbohydrates and cholesterol, you can choose from the three approaches: the Carbohydrate Strategy, the Cholesterol Strategy, or the Combined Strategy. This chapter describes them briefly.

- If you have purely a carbohydrate problem—that is, if you have signs of insulin resistance and you do not have high blood levels of bad cholesterol—you should follow the Carbohydrate Strategy.

- If you have purely a cholesterol problem—that is, you have high blood levels of bad cholesterol but no signs of insulin resistance—you should follow the Cholesterol Strategy.

- If you have both problems, you should follow the Combined Strategy.

PART 3
CUSTOM-DESIGNING YOUR DIET TO YOUR METABOLISM

So, you want to lose weight and get healthier. And, you would really love to quit obsessing about having a heart attack or developing diabetes (especially if you have a genetic proclivity for diabetes or heart disease, making that legacy never far from your mind). And you've just discovered a refreshingly hopeful message in *The New Low-Carb Way*—that losing weight and getting in charge of your health requires nothing more than tweaking your diet and exercise plans to fit your particular body-chemistry profile. This is exciting news because it means you have to make only minor changes that you can live with for the rest of your life, not just for a month or two of "going on a diet."

Part 3 starts with a look at how Americans got so fat so fast (chapter 9, "Why We Are So Fat: Thirty Years of Carbing Up") and moves on to explain how to reduce sudden surges of blood-glucose shocks, which aggravate insulin resistance and promote weight gain (chapter 10, "Avoiding the Aftershocks of Glucose"); followed by a detailed eating program in chapter 11, "Purging Glucose Shocks from Your Diet," and chapter 12, "Good Fat, Bad Fat, or Just Plain Fat?" and, finally, chapter 13, "The Secrets to Losing Weight and Keeping It Off."

CHAPTER 9

Why We Are Fat: Thirty Years of Carbing Up

Whatever is causing today's scourge of obesity started about thirty years ago, because before then, Americans were slimmer and fewer people had diabetes. The incidence of obesity was 13 percent, less than half of what it is now, and hadn't changed for years. But around 1970, the obesity rate suddenly started rising. What happened?

Some people attribute the change to America's rising standard of living, an abundant food supply, bad eating habits, sedentary jobs, not enough time for exercise, too much television. But all of these things had been around long before obesity in the United States started climbing. What has changed in the last thirty years is the composition of the American diet.

RIDING THE CHOLESTEROL-CUTTING WAVE

In the 1970s, public health agencies and professional organizations were confident that the way to prevent cholesterol from damaging people's arteries was simply to get it out of their diets, despite inadequate research to support that hypothesis. So, public health officials waged a war to reduce blood cholesterol levels and stem the rising tide of heart disease in the United States. They asked all Americans, regardless of individual disease risk or individual body chemistry, to reduce their intake of high-cholesterol foods.

For its part, the American public was receptive to any message that might help them prevent heart disease. Deaths from heart attacks had reached epidemic proportions, and people were worried.

Efforts by public health agencies to change the American diet coincided with a rise in the popularity of vegetarianism as an animal-rights and spiritual stance. The food industry also saw an opportunity to market low-fat, low-cholesterol products. In essence, Americans inadvertently became the subjects of a huge experiment on the effects of lowering dietary cholesterol on heart disease.

Around 1970, Americans started reducing their intake of fat and cholesterol and eating more refined carbs and sugar. Average fat consumption fell 15 percent. Annual flour and cereal consumption per capita climbed from 137 pounds per person in 1976 to 200 pounds in 1997. The average yearly intake of sugar went from 123 to 154 pounds.

The results? People kept on having heart attacks. Except for a decline attributable to a reduction in the number of people who smoked cigarettes, the incidence of heart disease was unaffected. However, the rates of obesity and diabetes zoomed to epidemic proportions, especially among the young.

Researchers learned something important: when you tell people to eat less fat and cholesterol, they become fat and diabetic.

Facing the Futility of Low-Cholesterol Diets

When the nation's experts realized that low-cholesterol diets weren't as effective for preventing heart disease as they had hoped, their first question was whether such diets even affected blood cholesterol.

Carefully designed research trials found that professionally supervised low-fat, low-cholesterol diets could indeed lower blood cholesterol levels. However, under the strictest conditions, the average decrease was only 5 to 10 percent—not nearly enough. To put that in perspective, cholesterol-lowering medication can cut levels by 50 percent.

Individuals' responses to low-cholesterol diets were highly variable. Some people experienced large reductions, others none at all. For some, the diets actually raised blood cholesterol. Of course, the occasional success story fueled the notion that low-cholesterol diets were the way to go.

Even today, many Americans still don't get the message because they've been brainwashed by years of dietary propaganda. Most people continue to believe that meat and dairy products are what cause heart disease and that a low-cholesterol diet is a powerful tool for preventing it. I often hear patients say things like, "My father died of a heart attack at the age of forty-nine, but his diet was terrible," or "I smoke a pack a day, but I'm careful what I eat." The reality is, there's little difference in diet between those who get heart disease and those who don't, and attempts to reduce dietary fat and cholesterol are of little benefit in preventing it.

WHY WE GET FAT

People get fat when they consume more calories than they burn off. However, the question should not be, "Do we eat more calories than we burn off?" but rather, "*Why* do we eat more calories than we burn off?" Our bodies have weight-regulating mechanisms that are supposed to balance food intake with energy expenditure. What is suddenly throwing these systems off-kilter? Let's look more closely at how our diets have changed in the past three decades.

▶ **We eat fewer eggs, less meat, and fewer dairy products.** Dietary propaganda suggests that we're fat simply because we eat fat, that we're devouring too much red meat and dairy products, but that's so far from the truth it makes you wonder if we are being intentionally misled. According to U.S. Department of Agriculture data, the total amount of fat in our diets has fallen by 15 percent since 1970. Average beef consumption has declined 22 percent. The amount of fat we consume in milk has dropped 56 percent, and we're eating 36 percent fewer eggs.

▶ **We are eating more starch.** The most dramatic change in the American diet in the last thirty years has been in our consumption of refined carbohydrates. We're eating much more starch than we did prior to 1970. Grain products— bread, buns, rolls, cereals, etcetera—were our largest source of calories to begin with, and now the average person is eating 46 percent more of those foods than three decades ago. French-fry consumption has risen 130 percent, and rice intake, 300 percent.

Candy gets a bum rap. Average sugar consumption has risen 26 percent in the past thirty years, but not because we eat more candy. Candy consumption has remained stable. Sugar consumption is up among adults because starch consumption is up. Children are consuming twice as much sugar in soft drinks as they did before 1970, so their sugar consumption is even higher.

Why does sugar consumption go up when starch intake rises? Starch is tasteless. It is often sweetened to make it taste good. Consequently, we get more sugar in baked goods—buns, biscuits, doughnuts, cookies—than in candy.

When it comes to *glucose* consumption, the average American gets twenty-two times more glucose from flour, potatoes, and rice than from candy.

▶ **The type of fat we consume has changed.** Before 1970, we got more of our fat from meat and dairy products. Now we get it in baked goods—cookies, cakes, pastries, buns. Cooking oil and shortening consumption has risen 52 percent in the past thirty years. In other words, the fat we consume comes with exactly what we don't need—more glucose.

It comes down to this: if you look at the way Americans eat now compared to the way we ate in the 1950s and 1960s, when fewer were overweight or diabetic, the major change is that we now assail our bodies with more starch and sugar. What we know now that we didn't know then is that the more starch and sugar in the diet, the more obesity, diabetes, and heart disease.

SEEING CARB ADDICTION SOAR

Although the theory that carbohydrates are chemically addictive has never been proven, most authorities agree that something about starch and sugar encourages overconsumption. There is an explanation for the similarity of starch consumption to chemical addiction. When you're hungry, appetite centers in various parts of your body send messages to your brain saying they want more food. They don't just say, "Send food when you get around to it." They say, "Send it now." Because the fastest way to get food into your bloodstream and to your brain is to eat refined carbohydrates or sugar, your brain learns to associate such foods with instant gratification.

The problem is, although starch and sugar quell hunger quickly, the satisfaction doesn't last long. Refined carbohydrates are digested much faster than other foods, so hunger returns sooner. Calorie sensors in your intestines tell your brain when you have had enough food. Many of these are located toward the end of your intestinal tract. Because sugar and starch are absorbed in the first few feet of your intestine, they never reach those sensors.

In addition, glucose shocks cause insulin secretion to overshoot, so that blood-sugar levels fall too fast. This causes hunger to return quickly. This cycle is especially vicious if you have insulin resistance, which causes excessive insulin secretion.

Because eating refined carbohydrates allows hunger to return so quickly, starchy diets have a different rhythm from diets higher in fat and complex carbohydrates. Not only do they promote snacking between meals to relieve hunger, but they encourage overeating at meals to forestall it.

Knowing the Truth about Low-Cholesterol Diets

Americans need to take a long look at the implications of eating less meat and dairy food and more starch and sugar. Consider the following truths about low-cholesterol diets:

▶ A low-cholesterol diet doesn't lower your cholesterol enough to reduce the risk of heart disease.

▶ Increased starch and sugar promotes obesity.

▶ Obesity raises your risk of diabetes.

In the midst of an epidemic of type 2 diabetes, it's impossible to justify the large glucose loads that high-carb, low-fat regimens impose. The rationale that nutritionists used for recommending a low-fat, high-carbohydrate approach in a population at risk for diabetes was that the benefits of weight loss would compensate for the added glucose. However, such diets rarely produce permanent weight loss, so people end up as fat as ever, with starchier diets to boot.

But the low-fat diet is *politically* correct. Low-fat diets definitely resonate with many people's vegetarian and animal-rights convictions. And, advocates of low-fat diets take comfort in knowing they are doing the planet a favor. It's true, reducing intake of meat and dairy products is not only kind to animals, it's environmentally friendly. If we didn't eat so much meat, we wouldn't need as much land for grazing animals and raising grain, and there would be less pollution from animal waste. If you don't lose weight, you can console yourself by thinking of the advantages for the environment.

Someday we might succeed in circumventing evolution and developing a healthy diet that doesn't rely on animal products. But, for most of us, vegetarian diets are impractical, unpalatable, and, for all their inconvenience, have little health advantage over diets that include meat and dairy products. For the sake of our health, we need to be realistic about our biological endowment.

The truth is, animal products contain vital nutrients such as vitamin B-12 and iron that are difficult to get from vegetables. If you stop eating all animal products, you have to supplement your diet artificially to survive. Although that's easy enough to do, the point is, our bodies developed a dependency on meat that evolved over millions of years. Vegetarianism is an admirable moral and ethical conviction, but a healthy diet requires more than switching from a diet of meat to one of bread, potatoes, rice, and sugar.

Appreciating Your Meat-Eating Heritage

High concentrations of fat and cholesterol in the bloodstream are toxic to most mammals—as, in fact, are high levels of the other two major food types, carbohydrates and protein. However, millions of years of evolution have made Homo sapiens into elegant meat-eating machines. Like other carnivores, most humans are genetically endowed with the digestive and metabolic capability to consume copious amounts of fat and cholesterol and quickly clear them from the bloodstream without adverse effects.

Technically, prehistoric humans were omnivores—they nibbled on grasses and roots between kills—but for the most part, they were carnivores. (And they were voracious ones, it appears: forensic analyses of cave dwellings indicate that, when hungry enough, our ancient ancestors would attack and eat one another.) Ancient humans sometimes even passed up muscle meat for more concentrated sources of fat and cholesterol, like bone marrow and brain. Such high-fat foods provided the sustenance our ancestors needed to recover quickly from long periods of deprivation and store energy to continue their fight for survival. Of course, most cave dwellers died before the age of thirty, so it didn't matter if they had high blood cholesterol or not. Only in the past few hundred years have humans started living long enough to suffer the consequences of genetic defects in cholesterol metabolism. In industrialized countries, subtle metabolic quirks that were previously inconsequential now limit the life span of many humans.

WHAT IS THE RELATIONSHIP OF DIET AND CHOLESTEROL?

Although the tendency to have high blood cholesterol is largely genetic, diet does play a role—but not in the way you might think. Under conditions of semistarvation—in which humans often existed in ancient times and which persist in many third-world countries—average blood cholesterol levels are lower than those seen in modern industrialized countries. That's why people who don't have as much cholesterol in their diets have less coronary disease. The rich, varied diet that people in technologically advanced countries consume not only allows them to live long enough to develop atherosclerosis, but also predisposes genetically vulnerable people to the disease.

Although most people in industrialized countries are able to eat what they want and remain free of artery problems, those with hereditary abnormalities of the genes responsible for removing cholesterol from their blood develop atherosclerosis even when they follow what is generally regarded as a healthy diet. That's because the typical "healthy" diet—whether it's low in cholesterol, carbs, or both—doesn't approach the deprivation seen in countries with lower rates of heart disease. Voluntary dietary attempts may lower cholesterol a little—5 to 10 percent on average—but that isn't enough to reduce significantly the risk of heart disease. What's needed is a 20 to 40 percent drop, but such reductions are unusual without forced starvation or cholesterol-lowering medication.

KEY IDEAS FOR TAKEOUT

- About thirty years ago, the incidence of obesity in America suddenly started climbing and hasn't stopped rising since.

- About the same time, Americans started eating less fat, red meat, milk products, and eggs, and more "refined carbohydrates"; that is, starch and sugar.

- Excessive insulin secretion, triggered by starch and sugar consumption encourages overeating and promotes fat accumulation.

- America's recent epidemic of obesity was probably triggered by an increase in consumption of refined carbohydrates and sugar. Individuals predisposed to insulin resistance have been affected most.

CHAPTER 10

Avoiding the Aftershocks of Glucose

Carbohydrates are foods your body breaks down to glucose. There are two kinds: fruits and vegetables in their natural forms, and so-called refined carbohydrates, or "starches." Fruits and vegetables are some of our healthiest sources of nutrition, but the refined carbohydrates are trouble. What is it about these foods that makes them harmful?

Considering the fact that the body eventually breaks down both kinds of carbohydrates to glucose, what difference does it make whether they are fruits and vegetables or starches? There is a *big* difference. Scientists have discovered that the speed with which glucose enters the bloodstream is crucial to how carbohydrates affect the body. Too much glucose entering the blood too fast causes "glucose shocks"—sudden surges of blood glucose that require large amounts of insulin to process. Repeated glucose shocks strain the body's metabolic machinery and ultimately lead to obesity, type 2 diabetes, and heart disease.

BECOMING CARB SAVVY

Both kinds of carbohydrates consist of chains of thousands of glucose molecules linked end- to- end. The difference is that the carbohydrate chains of fruits and vegetables in their natural forms are extensively branched and tangled—like brambles—and are surrounded by walls of indigestible cellulose. The carbohydrate molecules in refined carbohydrates are exposed and lined up in long, straight rows, like railroad cars.

As soon as refined carbohydrates reach your digestive tract, enzymes attack the links between glucose molecules and immediately unhitch the "cars" in the "train," releasing large amounts of glucose into the bloodstream within minutes. Fruits and vegetables take much longer to digest. Tangling of the glucose chains, cellulose walls, and fiber interfere with the breakdown process, and glucose seeps into the bloodstream slowly, sometimes taking hours.

Fruits and vegetables are absorbed over the entire length of your intestine as glucose trickles slowly into your bloodstream. Starch and sugar are absorbed in the first few inches.

Feeling the Aftershocks

To study the effects of repeated glucose shocks, researchers fed two volunteer groups diets of exactly the same composition, except that the carbohydrates in one group were prepared in ways that slowed the release of glucose into their bloodstreams. For example, they fed flour to one group in the form of bread, which enters the bloodstream rapidly, and the other group the same amount of the same kind of flour in the form of pasta, which is absorbed more slowly. At the end of six weeks, the group that ate carbohydrates in the more rapidly digested forms had higher blood-glucose and cholesterol levels and worse insulin resistance than those who had consumed the same food in more slowly digested forms.

Here's another illustration of the same principle. Pharmacologists have developed a drug called acarbose, which slows but does not block the absorption of glucose into the bloodstream. Acarbose improves insulin resistance, lowers blood sugar, and results in weight loss. Again, changing the speed with which glucose enters the bloodstream, even if the total amount doesn't change, makes a profound difference in the way carbohydrates affect the body.

Glucose shocks are especially likely to cause problems in people with insulin resistance. They cause excessive secretion of insulin, raise triglycerides, lower good cholesterol levels, and increase the tendency of blood to clot. One large study of the effects of acarbose on patients with insulin resistance showed an astonishing reduction in heart-disease risk: Among patients with insulin resistance, slowing the absoption of starch with acarbose reduced the incidence of heart attacks by 47 percent.

AVOIDING GLUCOSE SHOCKS

In the past, nutritionists gauged the effects of carbohydrates according to their total carbohydrate content as determined by laboratory analysis and made no distinction between rapid and slow digestion. They figured, for example, that fifty grams of carbohydrate in broccoli must have the same effect on blood-glucose levels as fifty grams of carbohydrate in white bread. After they discovered that the body responds differently to various kinds of carbohydrates, they learned that the best way to predict the effects of different carbohydrates on blood-glucose levels was to give volunteers a standardized amount of the food in question and measure blood-glucose concentrations for two or three hours afterward. Researchers have now performed such measurements on hundreds of different foods.

These measurements make it possible to rate foods according to the size of the glucose shocks they produce. In the following tables, you'll see that the glucose-shock ratings of various foods are compared to that of thirty grams of white bread (a half-inch slice), which is assigned a value of 100.

But before you review the table, let me clarify something: Scientists who measure the effects of food on blood-glucose levels use a scale called the glycemic index to compare various foods. Because this measurement does *not* take into account serving size, it creates some puzzling results. For example, the glycemic index of raw carrots is higher than that of spaghetti.

Many people have become confused by the lists of glycemic indexes in some of today's popular diet books. I have seen people give up certain healthy foods because of them. In fact, researchers who study glycemic indexes caution against using these numbers without further refinement. They are supposed to be calibrated to the size of typical servings.

In contrast, the glucose-shock ratings in this book make excellent points of reference because they take into account glycemic indexes *and* typical American serving sizes:

Food Item	Description	Typical Serving	Glucose shock rating
Pancake	5-inch diameter	2½ oz	346
Bagel	1 medium	3⅓ oz	340
Orange soda	8 oz.	12 oz	314
White rice	1 cup	6½ oz	283
White bread	2 slices, ½-inch thick	2¾ oz	260
Baked potato	1 medium	5 oz	246
Whole-wheat bread	2 slices, ½-inch thick	2¾ oz	234
Raisin Bran	1 cup	2 oz	227
Brown rice	1 cup	6½ oz	222
French Fries	Medium serving (McDonalds)	5¼ oz	219
Cola	12 oz	12 oz	218
Hamburger bun	Top & bottom, 5-inch (diameter)	2½ oz	213
English muffin	1 medium	2 oz	208
Doughnut	1 medium	2 oz	205
Corn flakes	1 cup	1 oz	199
Macaroni	1 cup	5 oz	181
Corn on the cob	1 ear	5⅓ oz	171
Blueberry Muffin	2½ -inch diameter	2 oz	169
Spaghetti	1 cup	5 oz	166
Instant Oatmeal (cooked)	1 cup	8 oz	154
Chocolate cake	1 slice	3 oz	154
Cheerios	1 cup	1 oz	142

Food Item	Description	Typical Serving	Glucose Shock Rating
Grapenuts	1 cup	1 oz	142
Special K	1 cup	1 oz	133
Tortilla (corn)	1 medium	1¾ oz	119
Cookie: average all types	1 medium	1 oz	114
LAB STANDARD: White Bread	30 grams (1 slice, ½-inch thick)	1¹⁄₁₆ oz	100
All-Bran cereal	½ cup	1 oz	85
Banana	1 medium	3¼ oz	85
Apple	1 medium	5½ oz	78
Grapefruit juice (unsweetened)	6 oz	6 oz	75
Orange	1 medium	6 oz	71
Pear	1 medium	6 oz	57
Pinto beans	½ cup	3 oz	57
Pineapple	1 slice (3½ inch wide)	3 oz	50
Grapes	1 cup (40 grapes)	2½ oz	47
Peach	1 medium	4 oz	47
Kidney beans	½ cup	3 oz	40
Grapefruit	1 half	4½ oz	32
Table sugar	1 round teaspoon	⅙ oz	28
Milk (whole)	8 oz	8 oz	27
Peas	¼ cup	1½ oz	16
Tomato	Medium	5 oz	15
Strawberries	1 cup	5½ oz	13
Carrot (raw)	1 medium (7½ inch long)	3 oz	11
Peanuts	¼ cup	1¼ oz	7
Beef	10-oz steak	10 oz	0
Pork	2 5-oz chops	10 oz	0
Chicken	1 breast	10 oz	0
Fish	8-oz fillet	8 oz	0
Cheese	2 × 2 × 1-inch slice	2 oz	0
Butter	1 tablespoon	¼ oz	0
Eggs	Two	1½ oz	0

Food Item	Description	Typical Serving	Glucose Shock Rating
Margarine	Typical serving	1/4 oz	0
Lettuce	1 cup	2½ oz	0
Spinach	1 cup	2½ oz	0
Cucumber	1 cup	6 oz	0
Broccoli	½ cup	1½ oz	0

Steering Clear of "White–Light" Foods

Notice that refined carbs—flour products, potatoes, rice, corn—almost all have glucose-shock ratings higher than 100 and that most other foods are consistently lower. The glucose-shock ratings of meat, dairy products, green vegetables, and nuts are too small to measure.

You can see how easy it is to recognize foods with high glucose-shock ratings. They aren't hidden or disguised. They are, in fact, what most people would call "starchy" foods.

Note, too, that starch is easily avoided. You can have your burger without the bread, for example, or eat a cup of blueberries for dessert and pass up the blueberry pie. You will find a more complete listing of glucose-shock ratings in appendix 2. But, in reality, you don't need to carry a list of foods around to get the glucose shocks out of your diet. The problem foods are a snap to spot.

TAKING THE FAST LANE TO GOOD HEALTH

Diets full of glucose shocks are problematic, because they aggravate insulin resistance, promote obesity and type 2 diabetes, and set the stage for heart disease. Conversely, diets low in glucose shocks improve insulin sensitivity, reduce insulin oversecretion, reduce blood-glucose and triglyceride levels, increase good cholesterol levels, and protect against atherosclerosis.

The discovery that glucose-shock foods worsen insulin resistance and raise the risk of obesity and diabetes has profound implications with regard to public health. In the past thirty years, the glucose-shock rating of the typical American diet has risen precipitously, corresponding precisely to the epidemic of obesity and diabetes that has hit this country.

CUTTING CALORIES WITHOUT TRYING

When you make the switch from a high- to a low-glucose-shock diet, you can reduce your caloric intake *without trying or even noticing*.

Several recent studies—including two in medicine's most prestigious publication, *The New England Journal of Medicine* (May 22, 2003)—show that if you restrict your intake of simple carbohydrates, even if you consume as much fat and protein as you want and make *no* attempt to reduce calories, you will on average consume fewer calories and lose more weight than if you consciously try to reduce caloric intake by following a low-fat diet.

One reason for this is that high-glucose-shock foods trigger more insulin secretion than low-glucose-shock ones, and insulin is notorious for stimulating hunger, encouraging fat accumulation, and promoting weight gain. Also, foods that release calories toward the end of the intestinal tract stimulate cells located there to release satiety hormones, substances that curb hunger. Refined carbohydrates never get that far because they "short-circuit" into the bloodstream in the first few feet. If you switch to foods that trigger less insulin secretion and use the entire length of your intestine, you will eat less without even trying.

CONTRASTING LOW-GLUCOSE-SHOCK WITH LOW-CARB DIETS

Low-glucose-shock diets are very different from low-carbohydrate diets. A low-glucose-shock diet requires only that you eliminate refined carbs—foods with glucose-shock ratings of approximately 100 or higher. On the other hand, low-carbohydrate diets require that you reduce your intake of *all* carbohydrates, including fruits and vegetables.

A low-glucose-shock diet has the following advantages over low-carb diets:

▸ You will find that low-glucose-shock eating is simpler. You need to avoid only five foods: flour, potatoes, rice, corn, and sugar—and nature has even conveniently provided you a warning label: they are all white or light.

▸ Your meals are tastier and healthier. Because low-glucose-shock eating requires only that you reduce your intake of a few bland, un-nourishing foods, this regimen is tastier and healthier than a straight low-carb diet. Fruits and vegetables add greatly to taste and variety and provide important vitamins, minerals, and fiber. The truth is, most people can't stay on a straight low-carb diet very long because they get tired of eating nothing but fat, protein, and green vegetables.

▶ You are eating more naturally. Reducing glucose shocks mimics the way human beings ate for millions of years—before obesity and diabetes became epidemic. Our prehistoric ancestors ate plenty of meat and vegetation but rarely consumed starch.

ARE WE ALL POISONING OURSELVES?

Because the average person now consumes more calories than ever in the form of refined carbohydrates, it's not surprising that many of us—perhaps, to some extent, all of us— find ourselves genetically underendowed when it comes to handling such large amounts of sugar and starch. If more efficient metabolic pathways were needed, humans would not have had enough time to evolve them.

Type 2 diabetes is a good example of a common metabolic vulnerability to the harmful effects of simple carbohydrates. Indeed, the number of Americans with diabetes is rising rapidly, and, in many parts of the world, the percentage of the population with type 2 diabetes has grown along with increased access to adequate nutrition. For example, Asia's incidence has increased dramatically as the daily caloric intake of the population has risen. (It's a common misconception that rice has been a staple of Asian cultures since antiquity, which, if it were true, would suggest that these countries' current heavy rice consumption doesn't contribute to their rise in diabetes and obesity. The fact is, although Asians have grown rice for ten thousand years, they ate it only in small quantities until recently, because it took the introduction of rice-polishing machines in the early twentieth century for rice to become a staple.)

As with disorders of cholesterol metabolism, susceptibility to type 2 diabetes varies according to genetic stock and patterns of human migration. For example, more than 50 percent of Pima Indians in Arizona have diabetes. In the United States, diabetes is more common among Hispanics, Asians, and African Americans than among Caucasians of European descent. In general, the most vulnerable ethnic groups are the ones that have most recently gained access to abundant sources of simple carbohydrates, because these populations haven't had as much time to develop resistance to the harmful effects of those foods.

LOOKING AT OTHER CARB-RELATED HEALTH PROBLEMS

Refined carbohydrates can cause problems other than obesity, diabetes, and heart disease. Here are some more troubles people have that are related to excessive starch and sugar consumption:

▸ Tooth decay. The most common starch- and sugar-related disease is tooth decay. In industrialized nations with the luxury of good dental care, people don't regard tooth decay with the same degree of seriousness as diabetes or heart disease, but in other parts of the world, tooth loss is a debilitating problem. In some countries, overwhelming infection caused by dental caries is a common cause of death.

▸ Gluten intolerance. Another disease related to simple

carbohydrates is *celiac sprue*. Some people are genetically intolerant to gluten, a substance found exclusively in grains, and *gluten* damages their intestinal surfaces, often causing debilitating, life-threatening digestive problems.

Recent surveys have found that sprue is more common than previously suspected, and in some countries, affects as much as 1 percent of the population. The treatment is total avoidance of most grains.

Looking for a toxin in the food chain? You've found one. Refined carbohydrates are responsible for more medical woes than any dietary contaminant ever discovered.

KEY IDEAS FOR TAKEOUT

- Glucose shocks are sudden surges of blood glucose that require large amounts of insulin to process.

- Glucose shocks are caused by too much glucose entering the bloodstream too fast.

- Glucose shocks aggravate insulin resistance; strain the body's insulin-making mechanisms; and lead to obesity, type 2 diabetes, and heart disease.

- Scientists have developed a way of measuring the severity of glucose shocks caused by various foods.

- The glucose-shock ratings listed in this book reflect the propensity of typical servings of foods to cause glucose shocks.

- You can eliminate most glucose shocks by avoiding a handful of foods: flour, potatoes, rice, corn, and sugar.

CHAPTER 11

Purging Glucose Shocks from Your Diet

Starchbusting is the name of the game. You don't have to worry about mild-glucose-shock foods like apples, oranges, grapes, beans, peas, and tomatoes. Just like you always thought, most fruits and vegetables are good for you; they are full of soluble fiber, sterols, fatty acids, and vitamins that improve insulin resistance, lower blood cholesterol, and generally outweigh whatever potential they have for raising blood-glucose levels.

All you have to do is eliminate a few foods that have very

high ratings—that is, over 100—and you'll put a huge dent in your glucose shocks.

COMPARING OLD FOOD HABITS WITH THE NEW LOW-CARB WAY

You can see how starch busting works by comparing glucose-shock ratings of a person eating heartily but avoiding very high glucose-shock foods with one eating more typical fare.

Low-Glucose-Shock Pattern Glucose-shock rating			Typical Pattern Glucose-shock rating		
Breakfast:	Grapefruit	32	**Breakfast:**	Orange juice	68
	Bacon	0		Bagel	340
	Eggs	0		Coffee	0
	Coffee	0			
	½ teaspoon sugar	14			
Snack:	Latte	27	**Snack:**	Coffee	0
				Doughnut	205
Lunch:	Chicken Caesar Salad	0	**Lunch:**	Turkey sandwich	260
	Milk	27		Potato chips	77
				Cola	218
Snack	Mixed nuts	7	**Snack:**	Corn chips	97
Dinner	Green salad	0	**Dinner:**	Caesar salad	0
	New York steak	0		Spaghetti, 2 cups	332
	Mushrooms	0		French bread	284
	½ baked potato	82		Butter	0
	Butter	0		Red wine	0
Dessert:	Dark chocolate	68	**Dessert:**	Cookie	114
Total shock rating: 335			**Total shock rating: 2,022**		

The Bagel Effect

You can see how quickly glucose shocks add up when you eat starchy foods and sugary soft drinks. I call this the Bagel Effect because the glucose shocks in one bagel exceed those in several days-worth of fruits and vegetables. Knowing how this works makes eliminating glucose shocks easy because there are dozens of moderate-glucose-shock foods (with ratings from 50 to 100) but only a few high-glucose-shock ones (ratings higher than 100).

CHOOSING LOW-GLUCOSE-SHOCK FOODS

FOODS YOU CAN EAT:

Red meat	Eggs	Cherries	Cucumbers
Poultry	Salad dressing	Raspberries	Peppers
Fish	Nuts	Strawberries	Peas
Seafood	Apples	Blueberries	Broccoli
Milk	Oranges	Beans	Spinach
Cheese	Grapefruit	Lettuce	Tomatoes
Butter	Grapes	Mushrooms	Apricots
Margarine	Pears	Asparagus	
Mayonnaise	Peaches	Artichokes	
Sour cream	Plums	Cauliflower	

FOODS YOU SHOULD AVOID:

Bread (buns, rolls, crusts, scones, cookies, cakes, crackers, tacos, etc.)
Potatoes
Rice
Corn products
Breakfast cereals
Pasta
Cola and fruit juice
Candy

If you compare the lengths of the two lists, you'll see that if you don't have to screen out moderate-glucose-shock foods, you have a wide variety of things to choose from. Simply concentrate your efforts on eliminating flour, potatoes, rice, corn, and sugar.

Follow These Tips for Eliminating Glucose Shocks

As you seek to eliminate glucose shocks from your diet, you'll find that using these ideas will enhance your chances of success:

▶ **Don't try to eliminate starches entirely—just satisfy your craving.** We all crave something sweet now and then. Candy, of course, satisfies this urge—but so does starch. *Salivary amylase*, an enzyme in your saliva, breaks down some starch while it's in your mouth and releases a small amount of glucose. This stimulates the same taste buds as sugar.

Your craving for starch may be simply a craving for something sweet. But you won't need to eat a plateful of starch to satisfy the urge. If you hold off starch consumption until the end of your meal—make it dessert—and eat about a fourth of what is customarily served, you won't need much to satisfy your craving.

▶ **Make sugar your ally.** Even though you want to eliminate as much sugar from your diet as possible, you can still regard sugar as a friend. Sugar is four times sweeter than glucose. That means it takes only one-fourth as much sucrose to satisfy a sweet tooth as glucose. If your starch craving is really a longing for something sweet, sugar can satisfy it more effectively and with less glucose shock than starch.

Many advocates of low-glucose-shock eating (me included) encourage sweets in moderation. This means that you should eat only the sweets that contain very little starch; examples are semisweet chocolate and hard candy. Avoid flour-based confections such as cookies, cakes, and pies.

I recommend a small amount of chocolate—less than one hundred calories—once a day after a meal. You may find that being able to look forward to something sweet after a meal helps you pass up bread, potatoes, and rice. Chocolate has plenty of fat in it, but this isn't about fat. There's some sugar in chocolate but not much; and you taste every gram of sugar in chocolate because it's not mixed with tasteless starch.

▸ **Expect to spend more money or time preparing food.** When you're getting rid of starches, you'll probably spend more money on groceries, or more time preparing food (instead of eating out). But think about what you're actually losing—starch provides no flavor and no consistency, just calories. A low-glucose-shock diet requires only that you remove tasteless paste. The good stuff—fruit, vegetables, meat, dairy products, nuts, even some candy—stays. All you have to do is regain your taste for good food in its pure form, undiluted by starch.

This change in diet may cost more money and/or more time because starch is are cheap, and you may have been saving money by filling your refrigerator and pantry with bread, potatoes, and rice instead of fruit, vegetables, meat, and dairy products. Letting restaurants prepare meals for you saves time, but don't forget that all eateries want to make a profit—and they can reduce costs by feeding you starch. To eliminate glucose shocks, you have to spend more money on food or take more time in food preparation.

Basically, you pay now or pay later. Invest in your health today, and you make up the expense in reduced medical costs later.

▶ **Develop a daily rhythm.** Try to work with your body's internal clock. Hormone levels and brain metabolism fluctuate according to a twenty-four-hour cycle. If you follow a regular daily eating pattern, your appetite centers adjust to that rhythm and expect certain amounts of food at particular times of the day. If you miss a feeding, your stomach growls, and your metabolism begins to fall into starvation mode. Eat more than you are accustomed to, and you'll feel overfed, and your body will convert those excess calories to fat.

Develop a daily pattern and stick with it. Unless you are doing hard physical work, the rule should be two small meals and one big meal every day. For most people, that means a light breakfast, a light lunch, and a full dinner.

▶ **Eat breakfast.** Curiously, most overweight people don't eat breakfast. And that's the opposite of the way it should be, because breakfast, if it doesn't consist of high-glucose-shock foods, curbs your eating for the rest of the day. When researchers fed experimental subjects omelets for breakfast, these people consumed fewer calories per day than ones who skipped breakfast.

So, make a point of eating three meals a day. It gives your metabolic machinery something to work on and keeps it from slipping into starvation mode. When you skip meals, your metabolism slows down, and you overcompensate by eating more later.

▶ **Don't eat high-glucose-shock foods on an empty stomach.** Make your between-meal snacks low-glucose-shock. Even a small amount of starch or sugar gives you a glucose shock if you consume it on an empty stomach. Examples of snacks that won't cause glucose shocks are nuts, most fruits, vegetables, jerky, hard-boiled eggs, and cottage cheese. The time to satisfy a sweet tooth is after a meal.

TAKING SEVEN STEPS TO LOW-GLUCOSE-SHOCK EATING

In a low-glucose-shock diet, the few taboos are easy to recognize. Reduce the amount of bread, potatoes, corn, rice, and sugar in your diet, and you've removed most of the glucose shocks.

The following steps will help you reduce glucose shocks with little inconvenience and deprivation.

Step 1. Eliminate starchy entrees and fillers

You probably consume starch as entrees—pasta, sandwiches, pizza—or as fillers that accompany entrees—bread, potatoes, rice, french fries. Those fillers should be the first to go.

That doesn't mean you should eat less food. Just replace those fillers with other things—meat, vegetables, salads, nuts. Add a side dish of soup or salad, and push away the potatoes.

You may be wondering if you can get away with eating less starchy forms of the same food, like whole-wheat bread instead of white, or brown rice instead of white. In reality, all forms of bread, potatoes, and rice are bad. None of them has an acceptable glucose-shock rating. My advice? Try to lose your taste for these foods. It will happen if you let it.

The good news is that reducing your intake of starchy fillers is not a particularly awkward or logistically difficult thing to do. Look around you the next time you're eating with a group of people; you'll see some of them pass up the bread or push part of their potatoes aside. You aren't expected to eat all of the starch that's served to you.

Step 2. Choose beverages wisely.

Even if the rest of your meal is healthy, if you wash it down with cola or fruit juice, you get a glucose shock. Also, the calories in soft drinks *add* to rather than *replace* calories supplied by other foods. Researchers have found that when experimental subjects add *solid* sweets, such as jellybeans, to their diet, they tend to reduce their intake of other foods, but when they add the same amount of sugar in the form of a beverage, they continue to eat the same amount.

Here is a list of glucose-shock ratings of some popular beverages:

Glucose-Shock Ratings of Common Beverages

Cola	218	Cranberry juice	109
Orange soda	314	Orange juice	89
Raspberry smoothie	127	Grapefruit juice	75
Banana smoothie	119	Pineapple juice	109
Milk	27	Chocolate milk	82
Apple juice	82		

Here are some other beverage tips:

▸ Diet drinks are okay. They won't give you a glucose shock. However, they stimulate your taste buds and send false messages to your brain that food is coming, which stimulates hunger.

▸ Go easy on fruit juices. Most of these cause glucose shocks, but fruits in their natural form don't. The juicing process removes fiber and disturbs the fine structure of fruit, which raises its glucose-shock rating. You shouldn't drink more than six ounces at a time.

▸ Enjoy homemade smoothies. Blend fresh, whole fruit with milk or yogurt. Use no sugar and you'll have a delicious drink that won't cause a glucose shock.

▸ Drink coffee but understand that it can stimulate stomach acid and make you feel hungry. Don't worry about adding a little sugar. A potato releases more glucose into your bloodstream than do twenty teaspoons of sugar.

▸ Alcohol in moderation is all right. Red wine, white wine, and spirits add calories but don't raise your blood-glucose level. However, the nonalcoholic contents of many mixed drinks can. Beer and most mixers, including tonic and ginger ale, are full of sugar. One caveat: alcohol blunts the brain centers that tell you when you have had enough to eat, which means you are likely to eat more food when you precede meals with alcohol.

▸ Drink milk. This is an excellent beverage if you're trying to avoid glucose shocks. Fewer milk drinkers have diabetes and obesity than non-milk drinkers.

Step 3: Eliminate all breakfast cereals except 100-percent bran.
The glucose-shock rating of a bowl of 100-percent bran cereal is 85, which, unlike other cold cereals, isn't quite enough to give you a glucose shock. You may, however, push it too high by adding sugar, bananas, or raisins. Instead, add low-glucose-shock blueberries, raspberries, or artificial sweetener. Also, stay away from 40 percent bran or Raisin Bran, which are generously amended with processed flour and pack large glucose shocks.

Remember those Wheaties, Cheerios, and Sugar-Frosted Flakes commercials we were bombarded with when we were kids? Advertising told us that grain-based breakfast cereals were good for us, but they aren't, because they deliver huge sugar shocks. The glucose-shock ratings of most breakfast cereals—including Cornflakes, Grapenuts, Cheerios, Rice Krispies, and shredded wheat—exceed 125. Even oatmeal is bad. Its rating is 154, higher than Sugar-Frosted Flakes.

Unfortunately, many of us start each day by throwing our metabolism off balance with a big glucose shock. Mornings have become a time for grain products—cereals, toast, bagels, buns, and scones. Ironically, as maligned as the traditional bacon-and-eggs breakfast is, this is probably a better way to go. Start your day with eggs, breakfast meats, fruit, yogurt, or cottage cheese instead of grain-based items. (Cereal's only redeeming quality is fiber.)

Step 4: Add fiber to your diet.
Cereals with fiber, on the other hand, may be worth a slight glucose shock. Here's why:

▸ Fiber, the indigestible parts of plants—the skin, husks, and pulp—come in soluble and insoluble, both good for you in different ways. Fruits and vegetables are full of the soluble kind, but *insoluble* fiber is much harder to come by. In Western countries, the *only* good source of insoluble fiber is the husk of the wheat kernel, called bran, and the easiest way to get this is by eating bran cereal.

▸ Bran increases the amount of fat excreted in the stool, offsetting the calories it provides. That makes it the only common food that actually takes away calories.

▸ Lack of insoluble fiber is the only common, disease-causing dietary deficiency in industrialized countries. Inadequate amounts predispose people to irregular bowel habits and a number of aggravating digestive diseases, including irritable bowel syndrome, diverticulitis, hemorrhoids, and colon cancer.

Step 5: Reduce refined carbohydrates in entrees.

To reduce glucose shocks from starch-containing main dishes, eat fewer such entrees, and cushion the glucose shocks when you do eat them.

Here are some tips on meal timing and dietary approach:

▸ Reduce starch-containing entrees to twice a week for dinner and twice a week for lunch. For a week's worth of dinners, have pasta one night, a fast-food hamburger another, but for the rest of your evening meals, stick with meat, vegetables, eggs, and dairy products. For lunches, eat a sandwich for lunch one day, pizza another, and soup but salad on the other days.

▸ Eat your vegetables first. The order in which you eat foods is important in avoiding sugar shocks. High-fiber foods like salads slow the digestion of starch. In addition, delaying your starch intake until later in a meal gives your appetite centers time to respond to more slowly digested foods. It is a healthy habit to start meals with a salad. Meticulously avoid eating refined carbohydrates on an empty stomach. Nibble at starches and sugar only after you have consumed most of your meal.

▸ Deconstruct your food. Pasta dishes, sandwiches, pizza, and deep-fried foods contain lots of starch, so pick them apart. For example, not only can you bypass pizza crust, you can take it a step further—scrape off the cheese and toppings and eat them by themselves. You can significantly reduce glucose shocks by eating sandwiches open-faced, peeling off deep-fried crusts, and pushing starchy parts of entrees aside.

▸ Build a "starch pile" on your plate. Pick away a good portion of the refined carbohydrates, and place them in a pile along with some of the starchy fillers. Then, enjoy the rest of your meal. When you've finished eating the good stuff, you will find that the starchy stuff doesn't look as appetizing as it did at first. As you leave the table, you can take satisfaction in knowing that you avoided consuming an overdose of starch.

▸ Eat pasta al dente, with plenty of extras. I'll assume you're like me: you love pasta and don't want to give it up. But full of starch, and you should avoid it as much as you can. However, pasta has some redeeming qualities. Some kinds deliver less of a glucose shock than others, and there are ways to prepare pasta that can cushion its impact.

Your intestinal tract digests pasta more slowly than it does other kinds of starch. Flour consumed in pasta causes less of a glucose shock than similar amounts eaten as bread. This is especially true if the pasta is cooked al dente—lightly, to maintain firmness. For example, the glucose-shock rating of spaghetti boiled five minutes is 142, which is permissible, but the rating rises to 166 if cooked ten minutes and 213 after twenty minutes—enough to give you a large glucose shock.

Some pasta dishes are heavy with sauces of meat, vegetables, and olive oil, which is good, because the fewer calories you get from pasta and the more from other ingredients, the less starch you will be eating.

As a rule of thumb, pasta with meat contains about half as much starch *per calorie* as plain pasta. A half-plate of spaghetti with meatballs is as filling as a full plate of spaghetti alone but contains only half as much starch.

The table below lists glucose-shock ratings of various kinds of pastas. In general, the larger the noodle, the lower the rating. Note that gnocchi—a potato pasta—has the highest glucose-shock rating of all, with rice pasta running a close second.

Glucose-Shock Ratings of Pasta

Asisan bean noodles	118	Ravioli	141
Capellini	158	Rice noodles	181
Fettucine	142	Spaghetti, boiled 5 min.	142
Gnocchi	268	Spaghetti, boiled 10–15 min	166
Instant noodles	150	Spaghetti, boiled 20 min.	213
Linguine, thick	159	Spaghetti, whole-wheat	126
Linguine, thin	181	Tortellini	169
Macaroni, plain	181	Vermicelli	126
Macaroni & cheese, boxed	252		

Step 6: Choose whole-grain products if you have to eat baked goods.

Bread is such an integral part of American and European dietary tradition that saying it's unhealthy is almost a sacrilege. But, it's definitely bad for you. When it comes to causing glucose shocks, nothing is worse.

Most people in Western countries get most of their glucose shocks from bread. Ounce for ounce, bread delivers larger glucose shocks than pure granulated sugar. The next time you eat a slice of bread, think of eating a pile of sugar because it has about the same effect on your body.

If you want to reduce glucose shocks, you must reduce your consumption of breads, rolls, biscuits, bagels, cakes, pastries, crackers, and crusts. In those rare instances when you can't avoid them, choose whole-grain products. And by "whole grain," I don't mean "brown" bread but bread made of whole-grain kernels like cracked wheat or stone-ground flour.

Here's a list of glucose-shock ratings for breads. Notice that, contrary to popular belief, even most whole-grain products have unacceptable ratings. Although they release glucose more slowly than white bread they are heavier and contain more calories and carbs per slice. They do, however, contain more fiber.

Glucose-Shock Ratings of Baked Goods			
Angel food cake	216	Blueberry muffin	169
Banana cake	170	Carrot muffin	199
Chocolate cake	154	English muffin	224
Crumpet	148	Corn muffin	299
Doughnut	205	Scones	268
Apple muffin	107	Pancakes, white flour	346
Pastries	149	Pancakes, buckwheat	526
Bran muffin	149	Waffles	203

Cakes and pies, because they are flour-based and generously laced with sugar, are generally bad, but some are worse than others. Review the following list of popular baked goods. You may wonder why the glucose-shock ratings of some notoriously sinful delights are less than those of white bread. For example, chocolate cake—a synonym for self-indulgence—has a rating of 154, compared to 224 for an English muffin. That is because it's starch, not fat or sugar, that pushes the shock ratings of most baked goods into unacceptable ranges.

Step 7: Learn how to snack wisely.

You're not perfect. Occasionally, you're going to cheat, but if you're crafty, you can exert damage control.

Follow these snacking guidelines:

▶ Stay away from cookies, crackers, pretzels, popcorn, and candy bars (except those that are pure chocolate).

Glucose-Shock Ratings of Breads			
White bread (32 gm)	107	Croissant	90
Brown bread	124	Dark rye bread	114
Coarse, wheat kernel	213	Light rye bread	142
bread (80% kernels)		Bagel	340
Whole-meal barley bread	273	English muffin	224
(20% high-fiber flour)		Pita bread	189
Whole-meal barley bread	176	Sourdough bread	114
(80% kernels)		French bread	284
Oat bread	127		

▸ Eat nuts. These universally favorite snacks deliver no glucose shocks at all. In fact, eating nuts isn't cheating at all. They are rich in protein and fiber and won't raise your blood-glucose level. Stock your shelves with every kind of nut you like and reach for them whenever you get the urge to snack.

▸ Treat yourself to chocolate. The glucose-shock rating of two, one-inch squares of chocolate is 61, well within the safe range. It has sugar in it, but the sweetness is not diluted by tasteless starch. You get to savor it all. It also has plenty of fat, but if you're just trying to reduce glucose shocks, you don't need to worry about fat. A little chocolate after a meal—especially if it's semisweet—won't give you a glucose shock, and if the satisfaction prevents you from eating worse things, it's worth a few extra grams of sugar.

▸ Choose hard candy. You can savor all of the sweetness of

the sugar in it and satisfy your sweet tooth with an inconsequential amount of sugar. The only problem is that it stimulates your taste buds without delivering many calories, which stimulates your appetite. So, munch hard candy only after a meal.

▶ Treat yourself to some ice cream occasionally—it's not the worst thing you can do. Sugar and starch, not fat, determine glucose-shock rating, and although ice cream contains plenty of fat, some brands are acceptably low in sugar and starch. If you're trying to avoid glucose shocks, don't bother with *low-fat* ice cream or frozen yogurt, which have glucose-shock ratings as high as regular ice cream but aren't nearly as satisfying. Frozen tofu has one of the highest glucose-shock ratings of all.

LOW-GLUCOSE-SHOCK EATING ISN'T HARD

Be honest. Would you call reducing glucose shocks deprivation? Would eating a steak and a salad instead of spaghetti and French bread be unbearable? Would pushing potatoes to the side of your plate and having some chocolate for dessert ruin your dinner?

Low-glucose-shock eating is an intrinsically satisfying way to eat. You get more taste and texture from your food when you don't dilute it with tasteless starch. And you don't have to be a food expert to follow a low-glucose-shock diet. It's such a healthful and practical way of eating, you may not be able to find excuses for not following it.

Take the steps suggested and see how well your body cooperates. Unless you're a complete couch potato, your triglyceride level will fall, your good cholesterol level will climb, and you will steadily and comfortably lose weight at a rate of about two to four pounds a month—just enough to shed fat without slowing your metabolism. It works. I've seen it countless times.

Don't Neglect the Other Parts of Your Diet

A low-glucose-shock diet helps the carb side of your body chemistry, but what about the cholesterol side? If your body has trouble removing cholesterol from your bloodstream, low-glucose-shock eating *alone* may not be enough. You might need to modify your fat intake, and I'll show you how to do that in chapter 12.

Even if you don't have high blood cholesterol, it's important to have a dietary strategy that encompasses fats and carbohydrates. Changing the way you approach one part of your diet is easier and more effective if you have a good plan for the other.

KEY IDEAS FOR TAKEOUT

- The glucose-shock ratings of refined carbohydrates dwarf those of fruits and vegetables.

- The best way to reduce glucose shocks is to concentrate on those few foods that have very high glucose-shock ratings and don't worry about midrange glucose-shock foods like apples, oranges, grapes, beans, and peas.

- Concentrating on the very high glucose-shock foods makes reducing glucose shocks easy because there are dozens of moderate-glucose-shock foods (glucose-shock ratings of 50 to 100) but only a few high-glucose-shock ones (ratings higher than 100).

- The worst offenders are starchy fillers: bread, potatoes, and rice.

- Sweets that aren't mixed with starch, such as chocolate or hard candy, contribute little to total glucose shocks.

- The only cereal that doesn't deliver a large glucose shock is 100-percent bran cereal.

- All breads have unacceptable glucose-shock ratings.

CHAPTER 12

Good Fat, Bad Fat, or Just Plain Fat?

Fat has gotten a bad reputation, but the truth is, it can be good, as well as bad. Regulating fat intake is a part of most eating plans, and while low-glucose-shock eating doesn't require cutting out fruits and vegetables straight low-carb diets do, you may need to be careful about your fat intake.

Why? It's simple. Moderating your fat intake leaves room for fruits and vegetables. When you reduce starch intake, you can eat more naturally fatty items than you did before without actually increasing the amount of fat in your diet. Your diet may seem fattier, but it won't be, because you will no longer eating the fat that was in the starch you consumed. You'll be eating more items that are naturally fatty, such as meat, dairy, olives, nuts, and avocados, but you saying good-bye to all the butter, margarine, oil, and shortening that was added to the starch you were eating to make it more palatable.

Nevertheless, you don't want to go overboard on fatty food. Remember, it's not the increased fat that makes low-carb diets work. It's the reduced carbs.

REDUCING BAD FATS TO LOWER CHOLESTEROL

For weight loss, you should be concerned about the *quantity* of fat you eat. For cholesterol lowering, you need to control the *types* of fat you eat: saturated and unsaturated.

You can think of saturated fat as "bad fat" and unsaturated fat as "good fat." Saturated fat tends to raise cholesterol; unsaturated fat usually doesn't. In fact, certain types of unsaturated fat actually lower it.

If you have a high LDL level, you can sometimes lower it by reducing your intake of bad fat. Keep in mind, however, that this isn't for looks. LDL gets in your arteries. If you can find an eating plan that you can stay on forever that lowers your LDL, keeps it up. Otherwise, for the sake of your arteries, you're better off taking cholesterol-lowering medication.

If you're giong to rely on diet to control your cholesterol, you should check your blood LDL level regularly for years. One reason doctors bought into low-cholesterol, low-fat diets for treating high blood cholesterol was that back in the 1970s, when they started recommending those diets, it was difficult to measure good and bad cholesterol and triglyceride. All they had to go were *total* cholesterol levels. A month or two after patients started following low-fat, low-cholesterol diets, their total cholesterol levels often went down. However, total cholesterol includes the cholesterol in triglyceride. People with insulin resistance often have high triglyceride levels, and in these individuals, triglycerides temporarily go down during weight loss from any kind of diet. The reduction of *total* cholesterol doctors saw was often the result of falling triglyceride levels in patients with insulin resistance. The problem was, doctors didn't know about insulin resistance then. Weight loss from any cause would have produced the same results.

Don't Be Fooled by Early Success

It's important to distinguish the effects of weight loss from those of an actual change in diet composition. Cholesterol often falls precipitously while you're shedding pounds, but rises again after you reach your new weight. After a year or so, the average drop ends up being between 5 and 10 percent.

RESTRICTING SATURATED FAT

When low-fat diets succeed in lowering bad cholesterol levels, it's not the reduced cholesterol intake or even the lower total fat consumption that causes the LDL drop. It's the reduction in *saturated* fats. Where are you getting bad fat, and how can you get it out of your diet?

Saturated fats are ones that are firm at room temperature, such as butter and the fat that surrounds meat. Unsaturated fats, including olive and vegetable oils, are liquid. To lower your blood LDL level, you don't need to reduce all fats, just the saturated ones.

Reducing saturated fat and cholesterol is straightforward because, in the typical Western diet, most of it comes from two sources: the visible fat in red meat—the suet—and the fat in certain dairy products—that is, butterfat. You can get rid of most of the saturated fat in your diet by eliminating fatty cuts of red meat and high-fat dairy products.

Scrapping Suet

Although there is fat in the red part of red meat, it's different from the fat in the suet. It won't raise your cholesterol much. Contrary to popular belief, lean cuts of beef and pork don't raise cholesterol levels any more than chicken does. You can reduce your suet consumption by choosing lean cuts of meat and cutting away visible fat before cooking.

Ground meat usually contains generous amounts of suet, so if you're trying to lower your cholesterol level with diet, it's a good idea to reduce your consumption of prepared ground-meat products such as wieners, sausage, salami, pepperoni, and so on. Meat packers usually add a lot of suet to hamburger to make it juicy and to beef up the package weight, but you can ask a butcher to grind lean cuts of beef for you. That way, you know what you're getting.

AVOIDING BUTTERFAT

Americans get most of their butterfat from concentrated milk products such as cheese, butter, and ice cream. You can eliminate most of the saturated fat you get from dairy products by choosing low-fat milk, yogurt, and cottage cheese. These contain little saturated fat.

Although 1 or 2 percent milk has some butterfat, a glass or

two a day should not raise your cholesterol level. A recent study has shown that people who drink milk are less likely to have obesity and diabetes. Cheese is full of saturated fat. Although milk consumption in the United States has declined in the past thirty years, as Americans have gotten fatter, per-capita cheese intake has doubled. Cheese is a convenience food. It's an easy way to get the fat and protein we crave.

If you're trying to reduce the saturated fat in your diet, you should avoid butter. Margarines are mainly unsaturated fat, and at one time, butter lovers thought they were the answer. However, many popular brands of margarine contain a type of unsaturated fat called *trans-fat*, which behaves like saturated fat and raises cholesterol. Currently, the American Heart Association recommends margarine over butter but advises moderation.

You can now buy a butter substitute (Benecol) made from a type of vegetable fat called *plant stanols;* this product not only doesn't raise LDL, but it lowers it slightly—about 5 percent.

Palm and coconut oil are high in saturated fat, but these don't figure prominently into most people's diets. They are usually added to starch, so if you avoid high-glucose-shock foods, you won't consume much of these additives.

LIMITING EGG YOLKS

Advocates of low-fat, low-cholesterol diets usually recommend limiting consumption of egg yolks. The yolk of a hen's egg contains higher concentrations of cholesterol than any other common food; one egg yolk has as much cholesterol as a steak does.

However, as pointed out in chapter 3, dietary cholesterol doesn't affect blood cholesterol levels much. Your liver makes most of the cholesterol in your blood, and most of the cholesterol in your diet goes out in your stool. Your cholesterol level is determined mainly by how efficiently the LDL receptors in your liver remove cholesterol particles from your blood.

Nevertheless, excessive dietary cholesterol will raise your blood cholesterol if you also eat excessive amounts of saturated fat. So, unless your diet is very low in bad fat, you should limit your consumption of egg yolks. Egg whites and egg substitutes (Egg Beaters) are okay, because they are cholesterol-free.

SUBSTITUTING GOOD FAT FOR BAD FAT

In the past, advocates of low-fat, low-cholesterol diets suggested replacing saturated fat with carbohydrates, but now they are starting to recommend substituting unsaturated fats instead. These "good fats" don't seem to raise cholesterol levels, and some may reduce the risk of atherosclerosis by lowering blood LDL levels and raising HDL levels.

Knowing the Two Kinds of Unsaturated Fats

If you're trying to lower your blood cholesterol with diet, you should familiarize yourself with the two kinds of good fats: *mono*unsaturated fats and *poly*unsaturated fats. Monounsaturated fats lower LDL and raise HDL. Olives and olive oil, nuts, and avocados are good sources of this kind of fat. Many nutrition experts think that a good diet should include plenty of monounsaturated fat.

Polyunsaturated fats lower cholesterol, too, but have

some drawbacks. In their natural forms in fish, vegetables, and nuts, they're generally good for you. If they don't lower your cholesterol, at least they don't raise it. They also provide *essential fatty acids*—fats the body needs but can't manufacture. Nutritionists are especially enthusiastic about a type of essential fatty acid called *omega-3 fatty acid*, which is found in deepwater fish like salmon and mackerel.

The Downside of Polyunsaturated Fats

The problem with polyunsaturated fats is that they are *delicate*. Processing techniques can damage them and turn them into *trans-fats*, which behave more like saturated than unsaturated fats and may raise cholesterol. Unsaturated or not, the oil in many prepared foods and margarines, can raise blood cholesterol levels. Most dietary experts advise using vegetable oil and margarine moderately, even if most of the fat is polyunsaturated.

If you follow a low-glucose-shock diet, you don't have to worry about trans-fat. Most of the trans-fat in the American diet comes in starchy foods. When you get rid of the refined carbs, you eliminate most of the trans-fat.

Seeing Food Fats as a Work in Progress

Surely, replacing saturated fats with unsaturated ones could do nothing but improve your health, right? Don't forget that all fat, whether saturated or unsaturated, is high in calories. And, scientists have become less enthusiastic about unsaturated fats since they discovered that trans-fats raise cholesterol. Some nutritionists believe that too much polyunsaturated fat washes away valuable, harder-to-acquire omega-3 fatty acids.

Remember, while our ancient ancestors consumed oils in meat and vegetation, they didn't buy it in pure form by the quart bottle. Your body handles the fat in bulk oils differently from the fat in meat. Meat gives your digestive tract something to work on. Your stomach has to massage and soften the meat, and your intestine has to break down the fibers and emulsify the fat. Oils are more easily digested. Could it be that people are less likely to overeat fat in meat? I have encountered plenty of compulsive starch eaters, but never an obsessive meat eater. Several overweight patients have told me that they usually don't overeat meat because it makes them feel too full. Perhaps there's a message there.

Improving the Quality of Fats You Eat

Here are American Heart Association recommendations for reducing the amount of saturated fats you eat and replacing them with mono- and polyunsaturated ones:

- ▶ Limit red-meat entrees to two per week.
- ▶ Cut away visible fat from meat.
- ▶ Eat fish twice per week.
- ▶ Use ground sirloin instead of hamburger.
- ▶ Limit eggs to twice a week—substitute Egg Beaters or egg whites.
- ▶ Avoid wieners, sausage, salami, and other fatty ground-meat products.
- ▶ Limit cheese, ice cream, and cream consumption.
- ▶ Avoid deep-fried foods.
- ▶ Drink skim or 1 percent milk.
- ▶ Try to eat five helpings of fruit or vegetables per day.
- ▶ Substitute monounsaturated fats, such as olive oil, for polyunsaturated and saturated ones.

If you follow these recommendations, you should be able

to lower your saturated-fat consumption to a third of that of the average American. If that doesn't lower your cholesterol to safe levels within three months, the American Heart Association guidelines suggest that you consider taking cholesterol-lowering medication.

KEY IDEAS FOR TAKEOUT

- A low-glucose-shock diet removes the fat that is mixed with starch to make it more palatable. That allows room in your diet for more natural fats in the form of meat, dairy products, and oil-containing vegetables.

- If you're following a low-glucose-shock diet, avoiding going overboard on fat leaves more room for fruits and vegetables.

- The type of fat that raises cholesterol is saturated fat— mainly red-meat fat and the fat in dairy products.

- Egg yolks are full of cholesterol but raise blood cholesterol only if your diet is high in saturated fat.

- Unsaturated fats—the oils in fish, olives, nuts, and avocados in their natural forms—do not raise cholesterol. Some even lower it.

CHAPTER 13

The Secrets to Losing Weight and Keeping It Off

Every year millions of Americans go on diets, but only a few shed pounds permanently. Despite billions of dollars spent on low-fat foods and weight-loss schemes, the incidence of obesity and diabetes in the United States just keeps climbing. Nevertheless, some people succeed in beating their weight problems, so what's their secret? Do they have more self-control than others, or do they know something lots of other people don't know?

Researchers have never found any psychological differences between overweight people and those without weight problems. Although people who have tried diets and failed repetitively often become pessimistic about their prospects for losing weight, there are no noticeable deficiencies in willpower in other aspects of their lives.

After working with thousands of patients who were trying to lose weight and living vicariously their successes and failures, it's clear to me that those who succeed do so because they find the right strategy for them. Those who fail are usually doomed from the beginning by a flawed strategy, or if they find a good approach, they don't believe in it enough to follow it.

The advice I give here is based not only on my interpretation of medical research on diet, but also on experience I have accumulated in twenty-five years of practicing preventive cardiology. These are the strategies that I have found work best to help people lose weight, lower cholesterol, and prevent diabetes. New concepts about nutrition have bolstered my confidence in these approaches and have given me the incentive to share them with you.

LAUNCHING THE NEW LOW-CARB WAY

It's true—you really can *radically* lower your blood cholesterol level, attain a healthy body weight, and effectively prevent or treat diabetes, yet still eat the foods you love *in satisfying quantities*.

In fact, some of the things you'll do to make the New Low-Carb Way work for you are so easy that you may find it hard to believe they can make a difference. But trust me. Much of paving the way to better health has to do with rearranging your priorities, and the following guidelines will help you do that:

1. Delete the phrase "going on a diet" from your vocabulary. You probably think of "going on a diet" as a period during which you eat differently. You start the program when your enthusiasm is high, and continue until you achieve a goal. After that, you say, "Thank goodness that's over" and go back to your previous eating patterns, perhaps with slight modifications to maintain weight loss. Or, at least, that's the plan.

The problem is, it doesn't work. Ask any physician or nutritionist who has followed patients for years, and you'll hear the brass-tacks truth: if you reduce your caloric intake to the extent that you lose weight rapidly—more than, say, four pounds a month—the weight will invariably return. And, you don't just regain what you lost—you gain enough to top your previous weight. I'll say it again: *most crash diets not only fail, they make you gain weight.*

The reason crash diets don't work is something called *rebound.* Your body has a deep-seated survival instincts that don't care if you're fat; they just don't want you to starve. If you deprive your body of food, it will fight back. Within days, your body will go into a protective mode in which your metabolism slows to conserve calories. The problem is, your metabolism stays slow long after you go off your diet. Your body continues to burn fewer calories, so you gain weight eating less food than you did before. Typically, you quickly regain the pounds you lost.

But here's the worst of it: *the slowed metabolism persists after you regain the weight you lost.* Your body tries to store fat in anticipation of future deprivation. Not only do you gain back the weight you lost, you tend to gain *more.* The rebound effect leads to what's known as yo-yo dieting, whereby your weight bounces up and down. Starvation slows your metabolism, which encourages weight gain, which inspires another diet, and so on. But unlike a yo-yo, each time your weight goes up, it gets harder to bring down. Your metabolism slows with each cycle. Crash dieting, in effect, damages your body chemistry.

Since the starvation-followed-by-maintenance strategy leads to disappointment, why do doctors and nutritionists continue to recommend it? Unfortunately, people expect instant results, and doctors don't want to disappoint them by telling them it won't work.

But even if you're desperate to lose weight and willing to deprive yourself to do it, you shouldn't try to fight Mother Nature. Countless research studies confirm that the timeworn strategy of starving off weight quickly, then trying to maintain the loss, has *less than one chance in twenty* of working.

It's not that people can't lose weight. It's just that they persist in trying the same flawed strategies over and over again. But, there *is* a way to beat this problem. You can lose weight and keep it off permanently. And you can do it quickly by trying the New Low-Carb Way.

2. Accept that you probably don't have the willpower to make major changes in the way you eat. Who does? It's not that you can't change; it's just that you can't change as much as you wish you could. You misjudge your capabilities, reach too far, and fall short. Why not just try to accept the fact that you can only change a little? Face that you probably don't have the discipline to deprive yourself of good food for the rest of your life—and that's perfectly human and quite okay.

You've tried dieting. You mustered your discipline for a while, and perhaps you saw some results, but, deep down, you knew your old ways would return, and they did. Your weight bounced back up. Dieting didn't work then, and it probably won't work now. Why go through all that frustration again?

The New Low-Carb Way makes it easy for you to succeed this time without a major restructuring of your eating
patterns.

3. Face the fact you have a physical illness. If you're overweight, admit that you have a body-chemistry disorder.
Being overweight is a medical problem, not a character flaw.
Is it realistic to think that 64 percent of Americans have
character defects that keep them from satisfactorily taking
off excess weight? If being overweight were purely a matter
of willpower, does that mean that people back in the 1960s
(when fewer people were fat) had more character than we do
now? And if they did have that quality, why, around 1970,
did they abruptly lose it?

The good thing about a medical problem is that you can
get rid of what's causing it and cure it. However, you can no
longer regard being overweight as a harmless lifestyle choice.
You have to admit you're sick.

Don't want to believe that you have a problem? Look at
this fact alone: if your belly is sticking out—if you are in the
upper 20 percent of waist-to-hip ratio measurements—your
risk of developing heart disease in the next twelve years is 8.7
times normal. Your risk of developing diabetes is twenty
times normal. Why wait until you develop the consequences
of being fat to admit that your weight is out of control?

4. Identify what's causing your problem. Once you accept
that you have a serious physical condition, you start thinking
realistically. In that state of readiness, you can try to identify
what's causing your illness, and find a way to cure it.

If you fail to pinpoint what's causing your weight problem, you'll simply thrash around, unfocused. For example, if
you think your weight problem is multifactorial, or caused

by a psychological quirk, you are unlikely to change what caused it. Instead, you need to focus on the single most important thing that is throwing your weight-regulating mechanisms off-kilter.

First, check to see if one of the following medical conditions is thwarting your efforts to lose weight.

▸ Drug side effects. Some common medications promote weight gain; examples are antidepressants, anti-inflammatory drugs, and estrogen replacement therapy. If you're taking any of these drugs, ask your doctor to advise you on stopping or changing your medication. (Though estrogen pills are often blamed for weight gain, researchers who studied their effects on body weight found that after several years, women who took them had smaller abdomens, less body fat, and more muscle than women who didn't. The problem is that around menopause, which is when some women start using estrogen, they can gain weight whether they are taking hormones or not.)

▸ Low thyroid function. Your thyroid gland makes a hormone that regulates the rate at which your body burns calories. Reduced levels of the hormone promote weight gain.

But, if you're like most overweight Americans, you didn't get that way because of medication side effects or low thyroid function. You're overweight because you unwittingly bombarded your body with more glucose shocks than it could handle. And, chances are, you're susceptible to the effects of dietary starch and sugar because you have insulin resistance. It might be genetic, or it might be caused by being overweight.

5. Get rid of what's causing the trouble. You need to remove the problem that made you sick in the first place, and if you're like most overweight people, that means reducing the number of glucose shocks in your diet and taking measures to improve your body's sensitivity to insulin.

By paying attention to the glucose-shock ratings of the foods you eat, you can eliminate glucose shocks. The best way to improve your body's sensitivity to insulin is to activate your muscle metabolism.

Your body is designed for a certain amount of physical activity. Only in the past hundred years have people been able to avoid physical exertion to the extent we modern-day inhabitants of industrialized countries do. This near-complete absence of physical activity is a physiological aberration that has a lot to do with why so many of us get fat and diabetic.

But the kind of activity we need to restore normal carbohydrate balance is not what most people think of as "exercise"—it's *muscle activation* (see chapter 15). The intensity of physical exertion needed to make a difference is less than most people realize. It just has to be done right. In the next two chapters, I will show you how, with the least effort possible, you can turn on your muscle metabolism and regain your sensitivity to insulin.

The plain truth is that muscle activation is more important than diet for correcting insulin resistance and losing weight. And if you are impatient with waiting around for your low-glucose-shock diet to slim you down—if two or three pounds a month isn't enough for you—more vigorous exercise is the only way to quicken the process without slowing your metabolism.

You already know that exercise is good for you. However, you probably haven't tried a program designed specifically to reactivate muscle metabolism with an eating plan to eliminate glucose shocks. It's a potent combination.

ENJOY A NEW FEELING OF CONFIDENCE

Crash dieters often have an air of desperation about them, as if they know their house of cards is going to fall at any time. In contrast, people who lose weight by exercising moderately, cutting high-glucose-shock foods, and eating an otherwise varied diet, often exude confidence. It's as if they have discovered something wonderful. And they have.

You can experience this yourself, once you discover what made you fat and find an easy way to correct it.

KEY IDEAS FOR TAKEOUT

- Crash dieting slows your metabolism, an effect that persists for months after you stop dieting and practically guarantees that you will regain the weight you lost.

- To lose weight and keep it off, make small changes that you can continue for life.

- Instead of starving weight off, identify what caused you to gain weight and correct it.

- Certain diseases and drugs promote weight gain, but for most overweight people, the culprits are insulin resistance, sedentary living, and a diet high in glucose shocks. Correct the conditions that caused your weight gain, and you should lose weight steadily with little sense of deprivation.

PART 4
LEARNING
NEW MOVES

As a key part of the New Low-Carb Way, you need to move your body in such a way as to activate your muscle metabolism. This means that you will probably need to examine your conflicted feelings and slick excuses (exercise hurts, you don't have time, you don't want to bother, you don't look good in workout clothes) and decide that your health is more important than stubbornly continuing your slacker ways. In part 4, you'll see that the New Low-Carb Way doesn't ask much—just that you let your body activate its "muscle-switch," putting your metabolism into a smoother mode. It will take so little time, yet provide so many benefits.

CHAPTER 14

Practicing Exercise Reality Therapy

For millions of years, physical exertion was essential for survival. Humans had to roam, forage, and chase to live. Hunter-gatherers scrambled endlessly over rough terrain to forage for food and pursue game. Survival depended on their ability to ambulate from one place to another. Even as recently as a hundred years ago, people had to walk several miles a day just to accomplish what they needed to do to live. Then came the Machine Age, which introduced the use of coal, gasoline, and electric power and helped to reduce our physical workload. Mass agricultural production freed us from farm work. Mechanized transportation eliminated the need to walk anywhere but short distances.

For the first time in history, inactivity became an option, and today, large portions of the population rarely exert themselves more than walking a block or two or climbing a flight of stairs. Many of us ride to work in a car or bus, sit at a desk all day, and then come home and station ourselves in front of a television or computer screen.

SEDENTARY BEHAVIOR WILL SHORTEN YOUR LIFE

If high cholesterol and diabetes are diseases, then so is sedentary living. Inactivity sets us up for obesity, diabetes, high blood pressure, heart disease, anxiety, and depression. Today, the number-one cause of disability in senior Americans is leg weakness caused by disuse. Many elderly people have to use canes and walkers or live in nursing homes simply because chronic inactivity has weakened their leg muscles.

Although the rising rates of obesity and diabetes of recent decades correlate best with a rise in starch and sugar consumption, the gradual decline in physical activity set the stage. Living a completely sedentary existence makes your muscle mass decline, your carbohydrate metabolism fall out of whack, and your body lose its natural ability to regulate energy balance. You get fat, weak, and diabetic.

ACCEPTING YOUR LOVE-HATE RELATIONSHIP WITH EXERCISE

Aversion to exercise is a detrimental psychological quirk rather than a rational preference, which means you may want to take a close look at this universal human foible. As a child, you loved physical activity, but with maturity, you lost some of that unrestrained enthusiasm for running and jumping. Once you're grown, you decide that there must be a purpose for exertion—winning in competition, mastery of a skill, seeking adventure, earning a living, or improving health. You may still enjoy exercise, but you need motivation to do it.

Also, in midlife, some stumbling blocks to exercise crop up: your joints lose elasticity, and the bounce in your stride becomes more of a thud. Speed, balance, and coordination, though still serviceable, aren't as good as when you were younger. This decline in physicality may be hard for you to accept, which leads to focusing more on the intellectual and social sides of life—areas in which your skills are rising—and less on the physical side, where your prowess is waning.

Fine-tuning Excuses

When you want to avoid something, you become an expert at coming up with great excuses for not doing it. That's why, in my twenty-five years of medical practice, I personally have heard several thousand excuses for not exercising. The most common reason is lack of time. But if that's legitimate, how come younger people who are working their way up in careers and raising small children are more likely to set aside time for exercise than older, more established folks whose children are grown?

Clearly, a conscious or subconscious aversion to exertion, rather than a genuine lack of time, keeps some people from exercising. What's unfortunate is that this perceived lack of time seems to get worse exactly when people need exercise the most, as they age.

Another common excuse for not exercising has to do with aches and pains. One sore spot often provides an excuse for not exercising the others. Backaches and stiff knees head the list. In most cases, exercise is exactly what's needed.

UNLEASHING YOUR NATURAL AFFINITY FOR EXERCISE

The trick is to suppress your aversion to exercise long enough to initiate physical activity, and you'll find that a natural affinity for action takes over. And don't get discouraged just because you're sometimes hit with pangs of laziness when it's time to work out or walk. A world-class triathlete once told me that when he didn't feel like exercising but made himself do it anyway, he had the greatest surges of energy.

Taking Advantage of the Boost

Pre-exercise lethargy and postexercise exhilaration probably result from hormonal fluctuations. Mild versions of the same body-chemistry downswings that cause depression are responsible for many of the sluggish moods we experience, and that is when the hormone-stimulating, antidepressant effects of exercise provide the greatest boosts.

My own reversal of attitude before and after exercise often astonishes me. A pang of lassitude—even resentment that I have to exercise to stay healthy—descends upon me before starting. But this dissipates immediately after I begin, and within a few minutes my mood brightens. Afterward, I regard the experience as a gift and look forward to my next workout.

Getting Yourself out the Door

The trick is in taking the first step. Just putting on your sweats and sneakers can improve your attitude. Once you decide to go work out, you will find that the lethargy, negativity, and uncertainty dissipate, and energy and confidence flow.

Seventeen years ago, I watched my wife take her first step into the realm of exercise. Kathy was disheartened because she had gained weight and gotten out of shape when she was pregnant with our second child. About three months after delivery, her exasperation grew, and one day, in frustration, she asked me what she could do to get back in shape.

Kathy had been a couch potato for all of her thirty-five years. Raised in the southern tradition that girls weren't supposed to engage in sweaty sports, she had never exercised in her adult life and was disdainful of the whole idea. I told her that she might want to leave the house and go for a short jog—something she had never done in her life. She took my advice.

When she returned, her attitude brightened, and I never saw her so discouraged again. She discovered that exercise was the key to feeling good physically and mentally. After a few more jogs, she looked for a form of exercise she would find more enjoyable. She enrolled in an aerobics class, and now she has been doing high-intensity aerobics three times a week for seventeen years. It shows. She regained and kept her youthful figure, and she did it without dieting.

Staying with the Program

I was thirty when I took my first step. In the last years of medical training, I had let myself get pudgy and out of shape. One day, I was so disgusted with myself I decided to go for a run (in my street clothes since I didn't own a pair of jogging shorts). I could barely run a half mile—pretty bad for a thirty-year-old. But afterward I felt better, and I kept it up.

Running put me back in touch with the physical side of life. Later, I installed a chinning bar in a doorway and started supplementing the running with calisthenics. Eventually, I joined a gym. I do more walking than running now, but I have exercised regularly ever since. There have been periods, a few months or so, when other interests distracted me and I let exercise go. But each time I drifted away, I knew what I had to do to get back: *take the first step.*

You're the one who has to decide to take that first step.

Ratcheting Up Your Health

Regular exercise can relax you, invigorate you, and help you control your weight. In fact, there are numerous reasons that exercise (even walking just 30 minutes, four times a week) is a great contributor to good health. Here are some of them:

▸ **Exercise relieves insulin resistance.** Exercise offsets the adverse effects of dietary carbohydrates. When you exercise, your muscles burn glucose before it turns to fat. Insulin resistance improves for forty-eight hours after a single session of aerobic exercise. In addition, if you exercise regularly, the increased muscle mass and improved cardiovascular conditioning permanently reduce insulin resistance, promote weight loss, and reduce the risk of diabetes.

▸ **Exercise lowers your fatness set point.** Your body has several mechanisms that match your dietary intake to your energy output, and the higher the activity level, the better these balancing systems work. Regular physical exercise restores your body's ability to regulate your weight. When experimental subjects lose weight by reducing their dietary intake, their metabolisms slow, their appetites increase, and they gain the weight back. Conversely, when subjects are made to gain weight by being purposefully overfed for a while, once they go back to their normal eating habits, they usually return to their previous weight without trying.

Exercise is the only way known to lower your body's fatness set point. Unlike dieting, which slows your metabolism, exercise raises the rate your body burns fat even while you are resting. It literally makes you lose weight as you sleep.

▸ **Exercise reduces triglycerides and raises good cholesterol levels.** Because exercise burns off glucose before it has a chance to turn to fat, blood levels of triglyceride—which is simply fat in the blood—fall abruptly and remain low for several days after exercising. High triglyceride levels "wash away" HDL, the good cholesterol. By lowering triglyceride, exercise restores HDL and helps prevent atherosclerosis.

▸ **Exercise lifts your spirits.** It produces the same chemical changes in your brain that an antidepressant drug such as Prozac does, raising levels of a natural body chemical called *serotonin* that relieves depression. According to research studies, exercise cures mild depression as effectively as medication.

▸ **Exercise stimulates your endorphins, the body's natural painkillers.** These chemicals are responsible for the feeling of calmness and well-being that exercise promotes.

The Older You Are, the More Important Exercise Is

Before age forty, you can maintain muscle strength and endurance with minimal exercise. That's why younger people often appear muscular and capable of vigorous physical activity even if they don't exercise much. But as you reach middle age, things change. If you make no effort to maintain your strength, your muscles shrivel up and your endurance fades, and by age fifty, much of your muscle will have turned to flab. Exercise prevents or reverses that decline. If you engage in regular physical exertion, you can maintain muscle strength and endurance well into your nineties.

▶ **Exercise gives you energy.** It causes your nerve endings and adrenal glands to discharge adrenaline, which wakes you up, heightens your alertness, and gives you a boost of energy.

▶ **Exercise is a natural tranquilizer.** Because physical exertion discharges excess adrenaline, which accumulates with stress, you will feel calmer and concentrate better if you exercise regularly.

Antidepressant? Pain killer? Tranquilizer? You would think we would all be addicted to exercise. Exercise—like religious conversions, falling in love, or kicking addictions—changes people's lives. Not only does it improve your health and your looks, it restores energy and optimism. Some people are hooked on exercise, and they're healthier for it.

Simply put, your metabolism won't work right if you're a couch potato. Your body won't handle carbohydrates properly, your insulin levels will go up, and you will be at increased risk of developing diabetes and heart disease. And, no matter how good your diet is, you will have trouble losing weight. Lack of exercise is, indeed, a disease in itself.

If you cut out the refined carbs and get off the couch, you may be surprised at how your body starts cooperating. And, it doesn't take much exercise to make a difference. Research studies show that twenty minutes of walking four times a week markedly improves carbohydrate metabolism. Men and women who walk regularly are significantly less likely to gain weight or develop diabetes than those who are completely sedentary.

KEY IDEAS FOR TAKEOUT

- The past one hundred years is the first time in history that most humans have not had to exert themselves physically to survive.

- The lack of exercise that characterizes modern life is a physiological aberration that predisposes us to insulin resistance, obesity, diabetes, and a number of other medical problems.

- Exercise is a natural antidepressant, tranquilizer, stimulant, and painkiller.

- Most of us have a love–hate relationship with exercise. There is a natural aversion to it, but paradoxically, also an affinity.

- Inactivity worsens our aversion to exercise. Activity brings out our affinity for it.

- The way to overcome an aversion to exercise is to take the first step. Once you initiate activity, the antidepressant and stimulant effects of exercise overcome the lethargy-producing influence of inactivity.

CHAPTER 15

Turning on Your Muscle Switch

You don't have to be an exercise addict to reverse the effects of a sedentary lifestyle. The kind of exercise you need to lose weight and restore your body's sensitivity to insulin is *not* strenuous. I recommend two simple things: walk regularly and exercise your quadriceps. That's because you need both aerobic and anaerobic exercise. Activity that depends on oxygen delivery to muscles is called *aerobic* exercise. If an activity depends on stored energy in muscles, it's *anaerobic* exercise. (Think of "air"-robic as needing air, an-"air"-robic as not needing air.)

GETTING THE "SWITCH-ON" EFFECT OF AEROBIC EXERCISE

Aerobic exercise is important because it "switches on" bio-chemical pathways within muscle cells that put oxygen to work. This allows more energy to be produced, *relieves insulin resistance,* and, *when done frequently, promotes weight loss and prevents diabetes.*

The exciting news about aerobic exercise is that when it comes to losing weight, your muscles exhibit an on-or-off phenomenon. Just walking at a moderate pace for twenty minutes is all you need to switch on those metabolic pathways that burn oxygen and reduce insulin resistance. Exercising more than that burns off more calories but provides little added insulin-sensitizing benefit. Researchers have found that the improvement in body chemistry you get by going from being totally sedentary to taking a brisk twenty-minute walk four times a week exceeds the difference between being a regular walker and being a long-distance runner.

The Forty-Eight-Hour Exercise Rule

The beneficial effects of aerobic exercise on your carbohydrate metabolism wear off in about forty-eight hours. It doesn't matter if you run a marathon or go for a walk. In two days, the benefits are gone. You don't have to exercise intensely or longer than twenty or thirty minutes—you just have to do it often. The rule is, don't let forty-eight hours pass without at least twenty minutes of aerobic exercise.

Keep Your Body Switched to "ON"

While the discovery of the muscular on-off phenomenon confirms that frequent, moderate exercise is good for you, the point is not so much that exercise is good for you, it's that total lack of exercise is very *bad* for you. If you're not engaging in at least twenty minutes of moderate aerobic activity every other day, your body loses its sensitivity to insulin, you are likely to gain weight, and your risk of diabetes rises precipitiously. The message is clear: *nature abhors the couch-potato life.*

SIMPLE SOLUTION: PUT ON YOUR WALKING SHOES!

If you want to restore your body chemistry to the state that nature intended, all you have to do is what humans have done for millions of years: start walking. Walking provides all the exercise you need to switch on your muscle metabolism, put your weight-regulating mechanisms back into balance, and reduce your risk of developing diabetes.

Of course, any exercise that involves regular contraction of a large portion of your muscle mass will do the job. Running, swimming, and bicycle riding are great forms of aerobic exercise. But, when people middle-aged and older turn their lives around with exercise, they do it by walking, not by running marathons or becoming gym rats.

Tallying the Pluses of Walking

Here are several reasons why walking is such an important form of exercise for normalizing your body chemistry:

▶ **You'll like walking, so you will do it.** Most people find walking a pleasure. You get a break from your daily routine, and the exercise improves your mood and heightens your energy level. If you find walking unpleasant, it may be because you are overweight and out of shape, which is why you need to do it. However, the worse shape you're in, the faster your endurance improves. It won't be long before it becomes easier and you start realizing the benefits.

▶ **You get more bang for your buck.** Compare walking to doing biceps curls—lifting heavy weights with your arms, exercising muscles that are about the size of lemons. Your buttocks and leg muscles, on the other hand, are as big as soccer balls. Think of how many more calories they can burn by virtue of their size alone. Even though it takes some concerted effort to lift a dumbbell, the time your muscles spend actually working is less than a minute or two.

Walking is superior for improving insulin resistance and losing weight because the muscles involved are large and it's easier to exercise them for a longer period of time.

▶ **Walking is especially good for you if you're overweight.** There's one good thing about being overweight; you build strong leg and buttock muscles. The walking muscles of overweight people are generally larger and capable of burning more calories than those of thinner folks.

Also, being overweight is like carrying around a backpack. If you are thirty pounds overweight, walking requires almost as many calories as jogging would if you were at your ideal weight. The beauty is, because your leg muscles are stronger than they would be if you were lighter, the exertion won't seem as difficult.

Knowing Proper Technique for Health Walking

You want to walk to improve your health, right? You're not trying to win a contest, beat a speed, or do anything other than feeling better and alleviating insulin resistance. Consider the following tips:

▸ **Don't worry about building endurance. Just think about improving your body chemistry.** The *intensity* of exercise is important when it comes to building endurance. The faster you walk or run, the more stamina you will develop. But intensity isn't so important when you're exercising to combat insulin resistance, and lose weight. You can compensate for a lack of speed by spending a little more time doing it.

▸ **Go the distance.** It doesn't matter if you run or walk. All you have to do is cover the distance. Walking two miles will improve your carbohydrate metabolism and promote weight loss as much as running the same distance will.

▸ **Walk fast enough to generate some heat.** When it comes to activating muscle switches, you don't need to walk so fast that you get short of breath. A comfortable pace will do as long as it is continous. You should walk at a pace that generates some heat, and fast enough to feel warmer as you walk. You can measure your walking speed by timing yourself over a known distance. Table 15.1 lists optimum pace according to age.

Table 15.1
Approximate Walking Speed Needed to Achieve Metabolic Benefit

Age	Speed
Less than 40 yrs	4.0 MPH
40–50 yrs	3.7 MPH
50–60 yrs	3.4 MPH
60–70 yrs	3.1 MPH
70–80 yrs	2.8 MPH
80 + yrs	2.5 MPH

If you're overweight, you don't need to walk as fast as you do if you are lighter, to get the same amount of exercise. To determine if you're walking fast enough, take your pulse during or immediately after exercise. Table 15.2 lists target exercise heart rates according to age. Understand, too, that the maximum heart rate you can achieve during exercise declines steadily with age *no matter how fit you are*. In other words, don't try to match the heart rates of younger people.

Table 15.2
Target Heart Rates

Age range	For Improving Body Chemistry (Beats per minute)	For Improving Endurance (Beats per minute)
20–30 yrs	118	136
30–40 yrs	111	129
40–50 yrs	104	121
50–60 yrs	97	112
60–70 yrs	90	105
70–80 yrs	85	96
80+ yrs	80	90

An easy way to pace yourself is by timing each step. Count seconds by whispering "one thousand one, one thousand two," etcetera. Shoot for just under two steps per second.

▸ **Walk at least eight miles a week.** The *minimum* amount of walking needed to improve insulin resistance and reduce cardiovascular risk is about eight miles per week. The optimum distance is about ten miles per week. You get added benefit when you walk more, but most of the good occurs in the first eight miles (Table 15.3).

Table 15.3 Walking Distances Needed for Health Benefits	
Less than 4 miles per week	Metabolic shutdown: muscles become resistant to insulin, blood triglycerides rise, good cholesterol falls, blood coagulates quicker, lasting weight loss unlikely.
4–10 miles per week	Improved insulin sensitivity, lower triglycerides, blood clots prevented, antidepressant effects, lasting weight loss possible.
More than 10 miles per week	Noticeable improvement in endurance, lasting weight loss likely.

BUILDING YOUR QUADS

Although you can get most of the body-chemistry benefits of exercise just by walking, you will be richly rewarded for your effort if you add one more step to your exercise regimen: building up your thigh muscles—your *quadriceps*.

Even though your quads are important for walking, walking doesn't strengthen them much. It does toughen up the muscles that propel you—your hamstring and buttocks muscles—but your quadriceps get less benefit. That's why you need to have a plan for strengthening your quadriceps even if you're already a good walker. This is where the concept of anaerobic exercise comes in.

In lifting a weight, the effort is intense but brief. It uses energy stored in the muscles but doesn't last long enough to require your heart and lungs to deliver more oxygen. Your muscle energy stores are replenished after the exertion is over. Brief exertion, even though strenuous, doesn't exercise your heart or lungs as much as aerobic activity does and is less effective at alleviating insulin sensitivity. But here's the trick: anaerobic exercise is much better than aerobic exercise for strengthening muscles. The more muscular force an activity requires, the more effective it is at strengthening muscles.

You don't need to weight train for as long or as often as you need to do aerobic exercise. Just two 5- or 10-minute sessions per week of weight training can strengthen your muscles if the force you generate is near your maximal effort.

The best way to strengthen your quadriceps is to push against heavy resistance with your legs. You need to strain hard, but you don't have to do it for very long. Climbing hills or stairs is good quad-strengthening exercise. Exercise equipment specifically designed for this purpose is very effective. Just keep in mind the difference between aerobic and anaerobic exercise. Spinning the pedals of an exercise bike for fifteen or twenty minutes against light resistance may be good for your heart and lungs, but it doesn't strengthen your muscles very much. Pedaling against heavy resistance, even if it's only for a minute or two, is much better muscle-strengthening exercise.

Understanding the Importance of Strong Quads

Here's why you should add quad-strengthening exercises to your fitness regimen:

▶ **Your quadriceps muscles give you balance and shock absorption.** The frailest older people can walk, as long as someone helps them to their feet and keeps them from tipping over. Their buttocks and hamstring muscles can usually propel them, but they often can't rise to a standing position or maintain their balance. Why? Their quads have weakened.

▶ **You will be able to live independently much longer than someone with weak quads will.** One of the best ways to predict if a person can live independently is to test quadriceps strength. If someone can't rise from a chair without using his or her arms to push up, the odds of having a serious fall or needing a nursing home in the next few years rise precipitously.

▶ **With strong quads, you add a spring to your step and improve your balance, which will make you walk more.** Although your quadriceps muscles are *not* the main source of power for walking, they are important because they provide balance and shock absorption. Weak quadriceps make your gait wobbly and stiff. Strong thigh muscles give your gait a solid, balanced feeling; add spring to your step; and make walking more pleasant. And the more you enjoy it, the more actively you will pursue it.

Start Working Your Legs at Any Age

You're never too old to strengthen your muscles. Researchers used gym equipment to attempt to strengthen the thighs of a group of nursing-home residents in their *late eighties and early nineties*. For two months, they did three sets of eight repetitions, three times weekly—about ten minutes of actual exercise per day. Amazingly, their leg strength increased, on average, 174 percent! Many of these seniors were able to discard their canes and walkers and ambulate independently afterward.

With such dramatic results, you might wonder why these folks hadn't discovered this themselves. Undoubtedly, they knew exercise was good for them. But the problem was, what led to their weakened condition was the natural aversion to exercise that comes with age and an environment in which walking was no longer necessary.

RECAPPING A SURE ROUTE TO WEIGHT LOSS

In a nutshell, here are the keys to alleviating insulin resistance and losing weight:

▶ Walk at the speed recommended in Table 15.1 for at least twenty minutes every forty-eight hours.

Losing Weight Fast

If you're in a hurry to lose weight, remember that cutting too many calories only slows down your body chemistry and sets you up for weight rebound. If you really want to lose weight faster and keep it off, there's only one way to do it: get more exercise. Unlike crash dieting, which slows your metabolism, exercise speeds it up. If you walk farther, add some hills or do some jogging, your weight will come off quicker.

A good way to enhance a walking program is to *walk-jog*—to run short distances during your walk. This interval training gets you into better shape than just straight walking, but it isn't as uncomfortable as continuous jogging.

The jogging part of walk-jogging may be easier than you think. One reason running becomes less enjoyable as you age or gain weight is that your joints lose their springiness. The tissues that connect your muscles and joints ache slightly with each step. However, nature has a remedy for this: *endorphins*, your body's natural painkilling, shortness-of-breath-relieving chemicals. Endorphins help ease the mild joint discomfort and breathlessness you experience when jogging.

If you run for a minute or two, your endorphins will start flowing. If you stop running, walk a few minutes, and start running again, the endorphins will still be there. You will probably find that your gait feels springier and your breathing more comfortable than you expected.

When it comes to burning calories and revving up metabolism, there is nothing magic about continuous running compared to walking and walk-jogging. You burn almost as many calories and increase your insulin sensitivity almost as much by walking as by running; it just takes longer to do it. Walk-jogging is almost as good for you as continuous running, but much easier.

▶ Cut down on flour products, potatoes, corn, sugar, and rice.

Sound simple? It is. This is enough for you to make significant strides toward returning your body chemistry to its natural state. Get ready to watch your blood-triglyceride level drop and your good cholesterol and energy levels rise, and see your weight fall steadily and effortlessly.

PUTTING THIS PROGRAM TO WORK

Note how a few small changes affected the following people:

Gene, at seventy-two, is slim and fit, but he wasn't always that way. When he was younger, he was markedly overweight. At the age of fifty-two, he got disgusted with himself for getting out of shape and vowed to walk an hour a day. In three years, he lost sixty pounds and never gained it back. That was twenty years ago. He still walks an hour a day.

Joyce, a forty-eight-year-old receptionist, gained thirty pounds during her thirties. When her husband developed type 2 diabetes, she started limiting her starch intake, and her weight stabilized. But she couldn't seem to lose the excess thirty pounds. Then the county parks department built a walking trail near her house. The path was a mile long and ascended a hill. Without trying to restrict calories, she started walking the trail four or five times per week—one mile up and one mile down. In a year and a half, she lost twenty-five pounds.

Going for the Trifecta of Endurance, Strength, and Flexibility

Although aerobic exercise helps prevent heart disease, diabetes, and obesity, it's also a great idea to do some exercise for improving overall muscle strength and flexibility.

One reason that good muscle strength and limberness are important is that they make it easier to engage in physical activity. Also, keep in mind that muscle weakness—not diminished endurance—is the leading cause of age-related disability. Many oldsters get frail simply because they lose strength in their legs, a form of disability that's largely preventable.

Another benefit of strength and flexibility exercise is its potential to prevent injuries. Most orthopedic problems are caused by soft-tissue injuries—damage to the tissues that connect bones, joints, and muscles, such as slipped disks, tennis elbow, shoulder bursitis, heel spurs, and pinched nerves. These are injuries you can prevent with regular strength and flexibility exercise.

Some people worry that they will bulk up too much from strength training, but that won't happen. A few months of weight training will visibly increase the muscle mass of a teenager, but after age forty, your muscles won't get much larger with exercise. Strength training lends tone and definition to muscles, but you can be sure that you won't get bulky.

Do whatever it takes to get moving, but consider a balanced program that tailors exercise to your body's needs as well as to what comes naturally for you. If you engage in a particular physical activity regularly for years, your body becomes increasingly suited to it. If you cover long distances, for example, you become lighter and wirier. If you lift weights, you get more muscular. Ironically, people often prefer forms of exercise for which their bodies are already suited and often neglect ones that could benefit them more. Thin folks usually prefer running to weight training, and often let their upper-body muscles wither. Stocky individuals may build up arms and shoulders that are already well muscled when they should be slimming down with aerobic exercise.

The key point, though, is that any form of exercise that gets you up and moving is great. But keep in mind that there are three facets to conditioning: endurance training, strength building, and flexibility.

Susan, a professional nanny, had been markedly over-weight for years. At the age of forty-six, she got a job babysitting for a working couple who couldn't provide transportation. Each day, she had to walk a mile and a half on hilly sidewalks to get to and from their house. Without dieting, she lost thirty-five pounds in two years. (A one-and-a-half mile walk may not seem like much exercise, but it requires more work if you're overweight.)

Rob, a forty-five-year-old software programmer, had his wife drive him only part of the way to his office so that he could walk the remaining two miles to and from work. Without changing his diet, he lost thirty-five pounds in a year and a half.

It's clear that the weight loss you get from walking and cutting high-glucose-shock foods is slower than what's touted in the claims of fad diets—about two to four pounds per month. But this isn't crash-diet weight loss; this is quality weight loss.

KEY IDEAS FOR TAKEOUT

- Moderate exercise activates metabolic pathways in muscles that relieve insulin resistance and promote weight loss.

- More intense exercise, although good for strength and endurance, confers little additional insulin-sensitizing or weight-loss benefit.

- Whether exercise is moderate or intense, the insulin-sensitizing effects of exercise disappear after about forty-eight hours.

- Dieting slows your metabolism; exercise speeds it up.

- Walking provides more aerobic exercise with less effort than any other form of exercise.

- Walking is especially good exercise for people who are overweight.

- Quadriceps-strengthening exercise improves balance and comfort during walking.

PART 5
STAYING
HEART ATTACK–FREE

No one wants to worry about having a heart attack. Now, thanks to discoveries about artery disease and revolutionary medications, we may not have to. Follow the suggestions in this book and you can move that fear way down your list.

Part 5 includes: "Seeing How Arteries Deal with Cholesterol" (chapter 16), "Calling a Truce in the Battle in Your Arteries" (chapter 17), "Statin Drugs: Magic Bullets for Heart-Attack Prevention" (chapter 18), "How to Take a Statin" (chapter 19), "Is Daily Aspirin Therapy for You?" (chapter 20), and "Seeing the Pieces of the Puzzle Come Together" (chapter 21).

Seeing How Arteries Deal with Cholesterol

"**Y**ou're only as old as your arteries" is a medical adage coined in the nineteenth century that's truer today than ever. How long we live—and, more important, how long we stay healthy—primarily depends on the health of our blood vessels.

Arteries are resistant to infection. They practically never become cancerous. They don't break or wear out. In fact, they would be remarkably trouble-free if it weren't for atherosclerosis—the blood vessel damage caused by cholesterol (see chapter 3). And, atherosclerosis wouldn't be nearly the menace it is if it weren't for its tendency to affect the coronary arteries, the vessels that supply blood to the heart. Narrowing and blockage of the coronary arteries by atherosclerosis is the number-one cause of death of Americans and Europeans.

A number of lifestyle factors, including cigarette smoking, sedentary living, and obesity, raise the risk of atherosclerosis. However, in each case, what actually causes the damage is infiltration of arteries by cholesterol. Nothing will reduce your risk of artery disease more than lowering the level of cholesterol in your blood.

MEET ATHEROSCLEROSIS

Atherosclerosis begins decades before heart attacks or strokes typically occur. Pathologists have found streaks of cholesterol in the arteries of car-accident victims who were in their teens and twenties. Although it rarely gets bad enough in early adulthood to cause trouble, later in life the process tends to pick up speed. For people who are prone to atherosclerosis, artery narrowing and blockage can lead to organ damage by the age of forty or fifty.

Why Arteries Are Not Like Pipes

Comparing atherosclerosis to a slow, steady buildup of sludge in a pipe never fit with the facts. Early on, doctors knew that severely restricted arteries often stayed open for years, and they also knew that wide-open ones could suddenly and unpredictably block off. The disease just didn't act like a gradual, accumulative process. What were they missing?

Cholesterol is a normal part of blood—an essential building block for cell membranes, hormones, and other important things. However, under certain conditions—no one understands the exact trigger—it starts to seep into the walls of arteries. This is usually a harmless process that lightly coats a few arteries without causing problems, but when it gets out of hand in vulnerable individuals, it leads to artery narrowing or blockage and eventually damages vital organs. Tantalizingly, some people's arteries remain clean throughout life. However, in most people who live long enough, some cholesterol will seep into the walls of their blood vessels.

Because severely atherosclerotic arteries feel stiff to the touch, atherosclerosis is sometimes referred to as "hardening of the arteries." That term is misleading, because it implies that hardness is the problem. On the contrary, localized *softening* of the arterial wall is what causes the most havoc.

NARROW ARTERIES GOT THE ATTENTION

Atherosclerotic buildup is worse in parts of arteries that are subject to distortion and hydraulic stress, such as bends or branch points. When this buildup of fatty deposits concentrates in one area and is large enough to cause a discernible bump on the inside of the artery wall, it's called a *plaque*. If a plaque protrudes far enough into an artery channel, it can interfere with blood flow, particularly during times of increased demand. In the heart, this can result in angina— chest pain during exertion.

Because narrow heart arteries can cause bothersome symptoms and are easily visible on X rays, they dominated the attention of doctors for years and led them to make an assumption that set back progress. Doctors presumed, without proof, that the plaques that produced narrowings were the ones that later blocked off and caused heart attacks. They thought that these constrictions gradually worsened until they caused complete blockage. The risk of a plaque, they presumed, was simply a matter of how much it narrowed the artery. Tight narrowings were considered dangerous because only a small amount of further growth seemed necessary to cause complete stoppage. Minor narrowings attracted less attention, because doctors believed it would take years for these to progress to complete blockage.

The notion that the danger of atherosclerotic buildup was simply a matter of how much narrowing it caused resulted in the massive mobilization of medical resources; heart surgeons focused on finding narrow arteries and surgically reopening them. This approach was appealing because it is relatively easy to diagnose coronary artery narrowings—they interfere with blood flow during exertion, cause chest pains, and produce characteristic findings on treadmill tests and X rays. Doctors had the means in hand to find narrow arteries, and they had the tools to fix them, which made the dominant mentality one of search and destroy.

Consider this typical scenario:

A man goes to a doctor with a seemingly minor complaint. Before he knows it, he's in the hospital having an angiogram, an X ray of the arteries to the heart. It shows a 90-percent blockage of an artery in his heart. He ends up having emergency open-heart surgery. Afterward, he can't stop talking about his good luck in finding the problem.

"Thank God they found the blockage and fixed it before I had a heart attack," he says afterward. "Now I'm walking three miles a day, and the doctor told me I have the heart of a twenty-year-old."

This man assumed that his narrow artery was about to block off and that reopening it cured him, that good fortune—and, of course, quick thinking by his doctors—saved his bacon. Often the narrative is embellished with such colorful expressions as, "my heart was about to blow up," or (my favorite) "I was living at the foot of the cross."

Repairing Blockages Doesn't Stop Heart Attacks

The truth is, the artery probably would have stayed open for years. And while the operation might have relieved some bothersome symptoms, it would have, at best, played only a modest role in preventing future heart problems.

Unfortunately, misleading notions about cholesterol and blood-vessel disease abound—the result of outmoded ideas and doctors' tendency to oversimplify things rather than take the time to explain them fully. Such misconceptions would be of only intellectual interest if they didn't affect the way people get treated. Unfortunately, they often result not only in confusion and apprehension but also in inadequate or unnecessary treatment.

Make no mistake, artery-opening procedures have been a blessing for patients disabled by angina, who were able to get back to exercising and doing the things they wanted to do. But after two decades of coronary bypass operations and angioplasties, doctors began to realize that the campaign to hunt down and reopen narrow arteries was not such a winning strategy after all. They had higher expectations for artery-opening operations than just relieving chest pains. What they wanted most was a way to prevent heart attacks. However, these kept occurring despite doctors' efforts to bypass and pry open narrow arteries. Why didn't reopening narrow arteries prevent heart attacks? Basically, the problem was simple: doctors looked in the wrong place for what caused arteries to block off.

Superficially, coronary artery disease seems easy enough to understand: arteries plug up and damage the heart, just like blocked pipes, right? Wrong. Comparing arteries to plumbing is deceptive. Heart arteries don't act as common sense might predict.

We assume that a narrow artery left alone would act like a blocked pipe and just get worse. But if a surgeon removed the obstruction, the vessel would stay open for years. Such analogies are appealing, but they fail to reflect a murkier, more complex reality—one that will eventually reassert itself.

Arteries are not inert conduits, and the difference between arteries and pipes is the difference between effective and ineffective treatment of artery disease.

A DARING EXPERIMENT REVEALS SOME ANSWERS

In the 1970s, some astonishing revelations about heart disease showed doctors where their thinking had gone wrong. However, some mavericks had to break away from the herd to provide some answers as to why artery blockage was so unpredictable.

Physicians had always assumed that patients having heart attacks were too fragile to undergo any procedure that might irritate their heart. They considered it reckless to inject X-ray dye into the coronary arteries in the middle of a heart attack. Nevertheless, a forward-thinking team of doctors in Spokane, Washington, decided to X-ray the coronary arteries of a group of patients within hours of a heart attack.

Finding the Culprit Behind Heart Attacks

These doctors saw something they didn't anticipate. In every instance, it was not a severe narrowing that blocked the artery and caused the heart attack. It was a blood clot. The clots usually originated from an atherosclerotic plaque, but the narrowings created by those plaques were generally mild. Sometimes there was no discernible narrowing at all. Clearly, previous thinking had been wrong. Narrowings weren't the culprits. The real danger was small, almost unnoticeable plaques.

Why hadn't doctors noticed this before? For years they had done X rays on heart attack patients, but they had always waited a few days for the patients' condition to stabilize—too late to see clots. Indeed, when the Spokane team repeated their X rays a few days after the heart attacks, the clots they had seen earlier had disappeared.

A few years later, another group of researchers tracked down the X rays of patients who happened to have pictures of their arteries taken in the months before having a heart attack. They confirmed the Spokane team's conclusions. Most of the arteries that blocked off and caused heart attacks were not narrowed much beforehand. The average reduction in cross-sectional diameter before the heart attacks was in the range of 40 to 60 percent, not enough to interfere with blood flow even during exertion. Sometimes, the offending plaque was undetectable with X rays.

Let me clarify something. Although small plaques trigger most heart attacks, severe narrowings are, in fact, somewhat more prone to blockage. Choke points in arteries aren't necessarily a good sign. The reason so many heart attacks are caused by mild narrowings is simply that they are more numerous. In a typical diseased artery, there are, perhaps, ten or twenty mild narrowings for every severe one. By virtue of their numbers alone, they're more likely to be responsible for blockage.

There's another reason small plaques are more dangerous

than doctors originally thought. Interference of blood flow to part of the heart stimulates nearby arteries to sprout new blood vessels that grow into the deficient area. This provides alternate routes of blood supply, which protect the heart during blockage. But if a narrowing is so mild that it doesn't interfere with blood flow, it provides no stimulus for new vessels to grow. If it suddenly blocks off, the damage is worse, because there are fewer alternate routes of blood supply.

LET'S HEAR IT FOR BLOOD THINNERS AND CLOT BUSTERS

When researchers discovered that heart attacks are caused by clots rather than narrowed arteries, they had made a major step toward preventing heart attacks. If they could stop the clots, they could avert heart attacks. This gave rise to the discovery that aspirin, a drug that inhibits blood clotting, is an effective way to reduce the risk of heart attacks.

The discovery that heart attacks are caused by blood clots rather than progressive choking-off of arteries rejuvenated interest in drugs to dissolve clots *after* they have formed. Cardiologists resurrected a 1950s-era clot buster called *streptokinase* and began giving it to patients with heart attacks. When patients got streptokinase within three or four hours of the onset of a heart attack, they improved dramatically. And, as you might expect, when doctors took X rays after the clot had dissolved, the narrowing underlying the blockage was often quite mild. Usually, the plaques didn't interfere with blood flow at all.

Taking medication to inhibit blood clotting is a useful strategy, but there's a problem: you need your blood to clot.

Potent anticlotting medication raises the risk of dangerous bleeding, and the kind of medication that you can safely take (aspirin) isn't strong enough to prevent heart attacks altogether. The forces that trigger clots often overwhelm the preventive effects of milder drugs. However, we now know that there is a better way to prevent heart attacks: stop what causes the clots in the first place (see chapter 17).

KEY IDEAS FOR TAKEOUT

- Heart attacks are caused by sudden blockage of the arteries that supply blood to the heart muscle.

- Blood clots—not gradual narrowing—cause blockages.

- Both large and small atherosclerotic plaques give rise to blood clots.

- Because small plaques are so numerous and often invisible on X rays, doctors cannot predict when and where a clot will strike.

- Coronary artery bypass operations and angioplasty can open up narrowings but cannot prevent heart attacks.

CHAPTER 17

Calling a Truce in the Battle in Your Arteries

When researchers discovered that clots rather than progressive artery narrowing cause heart attacks, they were puzzled. Why would a clot suddenly crop up in a wide-open artery? To answer that question, they started looking more closely inside the walls of arteries that had blocked off. What they learned was that cholesterol buildup wasn't the quiet, accumulative process they had thought it was. Cholesterol infiltration doesn't go unchallenged—the body fights it. In fact, collateral damage from the ensuing battle—not cholesterol buildup per se—is what makes coronary disease so unpredictable, so dangerous, and, ironically, *so treatable.*

SEEING HOW TROUBLE UNFOLDS

When cholesterol seeps into the walls of an artery, scavenger cells—called *macrophages*—move in from the bloodstream to remove the offending substance, as they would other foreign invaders like viruses or bacteria. Normally, when scavenger cells encounter adversaries, they secrete destructive enzymes designed to dissolve holes in enemy armor. Although those erosive substances are good at killing germs, they don't do much to cholesterol. The macrophages keep secreting them, but cholesterol remains unfazed. Eventually, the enzymes start dissolving holes in the plaque, and that is a problem. These holes don't heal normally. Instead of mending over with scar tissue, they fill up with a mixture of cholesterol and fragments of dead macrophages called *atherosclerotic gruel*. This stuff has the consistency of toothpaste or soft cheese. It inhibits normal healing and, because it has no structural strength, weakens plaques.

If plaque erosion gets intense enough, smaller pools of atherosclerotic gruel coalesce into larger ones and finally into a single large core. Although only about one in ten plaques has this boil-like structure, these are the ones that can cause trouble. Like boils, these gruel-filled pockets tend to burst, and that's what ultimately causes artery blockage. Here's how.

EXAMINING OVERZEALOUS CLOTTING

When a weakened plaque ruptures, it tears the inner lining of the artery. This would be harmless enough if it weren't for the body's attempt to fix the damage. Coagulation mechanisms respond to such tears as they would to any wound. Clot-forming cells in the blood, called *platelets*, spring into action. They cling to the damaged area, clump together, and within a few minutes form a patch to cover the tear.

But here's the problem: it would be fine if the platelet patch were shaped in such a way as to conform to the contour of the vessel wall, like a patch on a pair of trousers, but the clot is a formless blob, which causes trouble. Owing to its cumbersome shape and excessive bulk, it not only covers the tear, but sometimes plugs the artery entirely. That is how arteries go from being wide open to completely blocked in a matter of minutes.

Notice that artery narrowing per se plays no role in the sequence of events that leads to plaque rupture and blockage. Now you can understand why reopening narrow spots with surgery or angioplasty may relieve angina but does little to prevent heart attacks.

DISCOVERING THE CURE

About the time researchers were sorting all of this out, other scientists were studying the effects of a new cholesterol-lowering medication called *lovastatin*. Coming from the mind-set that artery narrowing is public enemy number one, they were anxious to see if lovastatin could reopen arteries, so they designed a research trial to test that theory. At the conclusion of the study, they were somewhat disappointed. Although the drug did a good job of lowering cholesterol, it had only a modest effect on narrowing. Two years of treatment reduced average narrowing by only about 3 percent.

Then they discovered something amazing. Although lovastatin didn't open up narrowings very much, the patients who took the drug had significantly fewer heart attacks than the ones who didn't. This was perplexing. How could lowering cholesterol prevent heart attacks if it had so little effect on narrowings? And if cholesterol buildup took place over decades, why would the medication have life-saving benefits so soon after starting treatment and so late in the course of the disease?

Although these findings were hard to explain in terms of the thinking at the time, they make perfectly good sense now. Lovastatin stopped cholesterol from seeping into plaques and inciting scavenger cells. Those cells, in turn, stopped secreting their erosive enzymes, which allowed plaques to heal and prevented them from rupturing.

REVISITING THE NARROW-ARTERY PATIENT

Remember the patient in chapter 16 with the narrow artery who thought that discovering and reopening it was his salvation? People who have had such experiences often believe—in fact, usually can't be disabused of the notion—that the artery would inevitably have blocked off completely, and that opening it up markedly reduced the odds of having a heart attack.

This is understandable. It's unnerving to find out you have a narrow artery in your heart. You imagine something closing off, like a faucet, with one twist of the handle left before it shuts off. You wonder, "What's to keep the narrowing from closing off altogether?"

Indeed, if atherosclerosis were a steadily progressive

process, narrowing would inevitably lead to complete blockage. The only way to prevent it would be to bypass or reopen the narrowing, which, if narrowing were a gradual process, would guarantee years of security against heart attacks. But that's not how it works. Coronary artery disease is unpredictable; it is characterized by years of stability punctuated by seemingly random artery blockages. The behavior of narrowings bears little resemblance to the image of gunk building up in pipes.

NARROWING DOES NOT A BLOCKAGE MAKE

Have you ever tried to stop water from flowing through a hose by stepping on it? It might narrow the channel a little, but it's difficult to block the flow completely. You usually have to pick it up and kink it. Similarly, artery narrowings resist blockage. Most never progress to complete occlusion. When a doctor discovers a constricted artery in the course of a routine office visit, it's impossible to tell if it's going to block off completely, no matter how narrow it is.

A rush to open up narrowings exposes patients to the risks of surgical procedures and diverts attention from what is most important, and that's correcting the high blood cholesterol and overly vigorous clotting mechanisms that cause artery damage and blockage.

And, doctors should discourage patients from assuming that they are as good as new after surgery. Indeed, after going through a major operation, patients want to believe they can throw away their pills, but unfortunately, atherosclerosis is never a matter of one or two narrow spots in an otherwise healthy vascular system. Even if all narrowings are successfully reopened or bypassed, a diseased artery can block off anytime. Unless something is done about the underlying process of cholesterol infiltration, plaque rupture, and clot formation, artery-opening operations have little effect on your chances of having a heart attack.

THE COMPLEXITY OF ARTERIES

Arteries can do mind-blowing things. They can remodel themselves to accommodate atherosclerotic buildup. They can spawn new blood vessels that detour around blockages. The blood that flows through them can deposit cholesterol or carry it away. Arteries can go from being wide open to completely occluded in a matter of minutes. Clearly, blood vessels are not inert tubes, and they bear little resemblance to the pipes in your house.

The difference between arteries and pipes is the difference between the old way of looking at coronary artery disease and the new way. Leading cardiologists describe this new awareness as a new paradigm in thinking about coronary artery disease.

But old ideas die hard. Doctors and patients alike often forget how complex and dynamic arteries are and revert to the plumbing mentality, which is a dangerous misconception, and simplistic thinking can lead to unnecessary treatment and missed opportunities for prevention.

NAILING THE ULTIMATE CULPRIT

Cholesterol. It seeps into arteries. It incites scavenger cells and provokes them to secrete plaque-eroding enzymes. It hinders healing and forms pockets under the artery's inner lining that rupture, activate clotting mechanisms, and ultimately cause heart attacks. Reducing cholesterol does more than slow a gradual buildup. Almost immediately, it pacifies scavenger cells, stabilizes plaques, and reduces the risk of heart attack.

Get the picture? It's all about cholesterol. If you have any reason to believe that cholesterol is infiltrating your arteries, whether the cause is high blood levels of bad cholesterol or low levels of good cholesterol, your first priority must be to stop it. That means lowering your blood cholesterol levels *not just a little but a lot.*

KEY IDEAS FOR TAKEOUT

- Atherosclerotic plaques rupture and trigger the blood clots that cause heart attacks.

- Scavenger cells in the artery wall secrete erosive enzymes to destroy cholesterol that has built up there. These enzymes only weaken plaques and cause them to rupture.

- Reducing blood levels of bad cholesterol pacifies scavenger cells so they stop secreting destructive enzymes. This quickly stabilizes plaques so they don't rupture.

- Coronary bypass surgery and angioplasty don't prevent heart attacks, because they do nothing to keep athero-sclerotic plaques from rupturing.

- The most effective way to prevent heart attacks is to lower blood levels of bad cholesterol with cholesterol-lowering medication.

CHAPTER 18

Statin Drugs: Magic Bullets for Heart-Attack Prevention

There's no question: the easiest and most effective way to break up the metabolic logjam that causes high blood levels of LDL is to take a statin type of cholesterol-lowering medication. If there were ever a magic bullet, this is it. These drugs have saved more lives than penicillin. But if you're like many people I talk to, before you started reading this book, you had never heard of a statin. If this is a cure for the number-one cause of death of Americans and Europeans, why weren't you aware of it?

CREEPING ONTO THE SCENE

When you think of a scientific breakthrough, you probably imagine a sensational event—a pivotal discovery embraced by a waiting world. But important medical advances don't always happen that way. They often proceed stepwise without attracting much attention. The development of a pill that could effectively lower high blood cholesterol was truly a medical breakthrough, and it spawned a revolution in medicine—although a quiet one—and provided astonishing insights into the mechanisms of coronary artery disease. But it took several decades for the story to unfold.

In the 1960s, when doctors began measuring blood-cholesterol levels, they found only a weak correlation between cholesterol and heart disease. Many patients with coronary disease had normal cholesterol levels, and most people with high cholesterol didn't have heart problems. Nevertheless, doctors kept pursuing the cholesterol link. Although study after study linked high blood cholesterol with heart disease, attempts to lower blood-cholesterol levels with diet or medication were minimally effective at best for preventing or treating coronary disease. What were they missing? Why couldn't they make the cholesterol hypothesis work?

STUDYING HEART-ATTACK SPARSE COUNTRIES

Epidemiologists—people who study disease trends of populations—got a clue about heart disease when they measured blood-cholesterol levels of people living in countries where heart attacks were unusual. Although cholesterol readings of Americans ranged around 220, the levels of inhabitants of countries where starvation and malnutrition were common averaged below 160. If the researchers defined "normal" as the average cholesterol reading for Americans and Europeans, most patients with coronary disease had normal levels. However, if they defined it as that of the typical rural Chinese villager, then most coronary patients had high cholesterol. In fact, people with cholesterol levels below 160 rarely get coronary disease, no matter where they live.

What was needed, then, was a way to reduce blood cholesterol to third-world levels, but for people with inborn tendencies toward high blood cholesterol, nothing short of moving to a Chinese village could do that. The standard low-fat, low-cholesterol diet lowered cholesterol only about 5 or 10 percent. Clearly, a stronger weapon was needed, something that would *radically* lower blood cholesterol.

But the cholesterol-lowering medications of the 1960s and 1970s didn't work very well. They typically reduced blood-cholesterol levels about 10 percent—not much more effective than low-cholesterol diets. However, they showed some promise. Combined with intense dietary treatment, they reduced the heart attack rate about 20 percent in five years, although the doses needed to produce such benefits often caused intolerable side effects.

Unveiling the Secret to High Cholesterol

In the 1970s, Nobel Prize-winning researchers Michael Brown and Joseph Goldstein unraveled the physiological mechanism responsible for high blood cholesterol. They found that the body has a powerful mechanism for clearing bad cholesterol from the blood. Tiny molecular structures on the surfaces of liver cells, called receptors, pluck LDL particles from the bloodstream and pull them into the liver cells, where they are broken down and metabolized. Genetic flaws in those receptors reduce their efficiency and cause cholesterol to back up in the blood.

The pharmaceutical industry used that knowledge to develop medications that could boost the activity of LDL receptors. The first drug of this type was lovastatin (trade name Mevacor). A few years later, several similar drugs arrived on the market, including pravastatin (Pravachol), simvastatin (Zocor), atorvastatin (Lipitor), fluvastatin (Lescol), and rosuvastatin (Crestor), all of which have generic names ending in "statin." Although these drugs vary in their potencies and durations of action, they all enhance LDL breakdown by the liver.

Instead of reducing cholesterol levels by 5 or 10 percent, typical for the old drugs, statins cut blood concentrations by 25 to 50 percent. One pill a day can make your cholesterol level look like that of a Chinese villager or, for that matter, a person with good cholesterol-metabolizing genes.

Finding Statins "Too Good to Be True"

At first, doctors didn't understand why lowering blood cholesterol levels could thwart heart attacks while having only slight effects on artery narrowing. They were still languishing in the plumbing mentality. They thought that *gradual* worsening of narrowings caused heart attacks. If lovastatin only opened up narrowings—and only after two years of taking it—how could it save lives so soon after treatment and so late in the course of the disease?

The first study that suggested lovastatin could prevent heart attacks had little effect on the way medicine was practiced. It was met with minimal fanfare among practicing physicians—certainly nothing like the media blitz that has accompanied other medical advances. Nevertheless, it presaged a revolution in medicine. Researchers began conducting larger studies specifically designed to measure the effects of statins on heart-attack rates, and they didn't have to wait long to see results. Study after study found that statins dramatically reduced heart-attack and death rates. One pill a day could reduce the heart-attack rate by as much as 75 percent. Benefits were seen in almost every type of patient—young, old, those who already had had heart attacks, diabetics, cigarette smokers, and even those whose cholesterol levels were normal to begin with.

WATCHING THE BULLET WORK ITS MAGIC

As time went by, doctors discovered even more advantages of statins, including the following:

1. Statins work fast. One of the most surprising discoveries was how quickly statins went to work to prevent artery blockage. At first, researchers were amazed when they found that the medications could prevent heart attacks after two years of taking them. Later trials showed benefits within a few months. Recent studies suggest that the drugs reduce the risk of heart attack within days.

How could statins work so fast? It's not surprising if you think about it. High blood cholesterol incites scavenger cells and causes them to secrete plaque-eroding enzymes. Reducing blood-cholesterol levels quickly placates these cells and stops them from secreting their enzymes, which stabilizes vulnerable plaques and keeps them from rupturing. After a few weeks, atherosclerotic areas become almost devoid of scavenger cells. Scar tissue cells then migrate into those areas, strengthen damaged tissue, and further prevent plaques from rupturing.

2. Statins shrink plaques. Although earlier studies suggested that statins had only mild effects on the size of atherosclerotic plaques, later research proved this impression wrong. These medications consistently shrink plaques.

The reason earlier researchers didn't notice that reverse remodeling had taken place was that they used *angiograms—* X rays of dye injected into arteries—to gauge the size of plaques. Angiograms outline the parts of plaques that bulge into artery channels but don't show how far they extend beneath the surface. Techniques that visualize entire plaques show that cholesterol-lowering treatment does shrink them significantly.

3. Statins improve blood flow. Statins not only prevent heart attacks and shrink atherosclerotic plaques, but they open up arteries and improve blood flow. Artery opening usually takes a few months and is more likely to occur with stronger doses of statins. After three to six months of vigorous cholesterol-lowering treatment, chest pains caused by narrow arteries often improve or disappear.

If you have narrow arteries, cholesterol-lowering medications may open them up. However, it may take a few months. In the meantime, you need to make sure artery narrowing isn't posing an immediate threat. Doctors usually recommend an exercise test to assess the risk. If you still have bothersome symptoms after several months of successful cholesterol-lowering treatment, and if these aren't satisfactorily relieved by antiangina medications, you might investigate the possibility of having an artery-opening procedure.

Nevertheless, the most astonishing benefit of statins is their ability to prevent sudden artery blockage. By reducing the danger of heart attacks, they allow time for the artery-opening effects of cholesterol-lowering drugs to work. Not only do these medicines save lives, but they make atherosclerosis a more predictable, easier-to-treat disease.

KEY IDEAS FOR TAKEOUT

- The easiest and most effective way to reduce blood levels of bad cholesterol is to take a statin type of cholesterol-lowering medication.

- Statins reduce blood cholesterol levels from 20 to 50 percent and reduce heart-attack rates by as much as 75 percent.

- After several months, statins shrink atherosclerotic plaques, open narrow arteries, and improve blood flow.

CHAPTER 19

How to Take a Statin

Besides being some of the safest and most effective medications commonly prescribed, statins—the amazing drugs used to prevent heart attacks—are easy to take on a regular basis. You simply take one pill a day. Side effects are unusual. You can expect to see your blood cholesterol level start to fall within a few days of starting a statin, but it usually takes about a month to see the full effect. If you stop the medication, your cholesterol will return to its previous level in a few days.

FOLLOWING SIMPLE RULES

The particulars of taking statin drugs go like this:

▶ You take a pill every day.

▶ It's best to take the pill at bedtime because your liver makes more cholesterol while you're sleeping than when you're awake. As a practical matter, however, it doesn't make much difference when you take your pill. If you have trouble remembering medication at night, you're better off taking it in the morning.

▶ You don't have to take your statin in any relationship to food. Statins don't counteract what you've just eaten or are about to eat.

UNDERSTANDING POSSIBLE SIDE EFFECTS

Statins are remarkably free of side effects, but you should know about possible consequences and understand what to do if they occur. Possible side effects are discussed below:

▶ **Rhabdomyolysis.** Rarely, statins can cause a type of muscle damage called rhabdomyolysis, which occurs in less than half a percent of patients. The symptoms are severe muscle pain and weakness soon after starting the drug. If this occurs, you should stop taking the pills immediately and have your blood checked for signs of rhabdomyolysis. The muscle damage of rhabdomyolysis heals within a few days of stopping the medication. However, there have been a few cases in which severe muscle damage caused irreversible kidney failure. If you have already had an episode of rhab-domyolysis, you shouldn't take these medications. There are alternatives.

▸ **Muscle aches.** Although serious muscle damage from statins is rare, mild muscle aches are more common. Such discomfort occurs in 1 to 2 percent of patients, and although harmless, it can be bothersome. Achy muscles are common even if you don't take a statin, so it is important to be sure the pills are the cause, not muscle strain or arthritis.

How can you tell if a statin is causing your pains? Typically, statins make the legs ache more than the arms and shoulders. Exertion often worsens the discomfort, which is sometimes mistaken for poor circulation or arthritis. Statin-induced muscle aches usually come on shortly after starting or increasing the dose of a statin, although some people take the medication for months before noticing them.

You can have a blood test for statin-induced muscle damage called CPK. If you're taking a statin and your muscles ache and your CPK is high—and everything returns to normal when you stop taking the medication—you probably have statin-induced muscle pain. Reducing the statin dose or switching to a milder one often solves the problem.

▸ **Headaches.** About 2 percent of patients complain of headaches, but usually, the problem doesn't bother them enough to discontinue the medication.

▸ **Liver irritation.** Like most medications, statins can irritate the liver, but this is uncommon and rarely requires stopping the medication.

On the up side, studies indicate that statins improve osteoporosis, a weakening of bones that occurs with aging. Evidence that statins reduce the risk of type 2 diabetes and Alzheimer's disease seem almost too good to be true. Studies are under way to examine these possibilities.

Deciding What to Do about Side Effects

If you think you're experiencing side effects to a statin drug, be sure they're caused by the drug and not just coincidental. There are alternative medications, but none is quite as effective at lowering cholesterol as the statin.

Here's what to do:

1. Stop the medication and see if the symptoms improve in a week or two. If not, the statin probably didn't cause them.

2. If the side effects go away when you stop the pills, that doesn't mean you should give up on the medication. If you can't take it, you'll miss out on the easiest, most effective treatment ever devised for preventing artery disease. So, for a week or two, take a break from the statins and then, under your doctor's supervision, try taking them again.

3. If the symptoms return, you can assume the medication caused them, but don't give up yet. Wait two weeks and switch to the lowest possible dose. If your side effects go away but the statin no longer lowers your cholesterol enough, your doctor can add a statin enhancer (see below), which will usually lower your cholesterol as well as will a full dose of a statin alone.

USING STATIN ENHANCERS

Small doses of other cholesterol-lowering drugs can increase the effectiveness of statins. If a full dose of statin doesn't lower your cholesterol enough, or if you can't take higher doses because of side effects, you may benefit from taking a medication to enhance its effects.

Statin-enhancing cholesterol-lowering drugs include the following:

▸ Niacin, a vitamin that can be purchased in any drugstore, can lower LDL and raise HDL levels significantly if you take it in large doses. The one annoying side effect is skin flushing. But a smaller dose of niacin taken with a statin can lower cholesterol further than the statin alone and without much flushing.

The flushing that niacin causes usually subsides after a week or two. Start with a small amount—about 50 milligrams—and wait until the flushing subsides, then double the dosage. Over a period of two or three months, work your way up to 500 or 1,000 milligrams, which are the doses needed to produce a significant statin-enhancing effect.

▸ Cholesterol absorption inhibitors also enhance the effects of statin drugs. Examples are cholestyramine (Questran), colesevelam (Welchol), and ezetimibe (Zetia). Cholestyramine is inexpensive but often causes constipation. Colesevelam and ezetimibe are expensive but remarkably free of side effects.

▸ Gemfibrozil (Lopid) reduces cholesterol production by

the liver and enhances the cholesterol-lowering effects of statins. However, it may aggravate liver irritation and muscle soreness.

All of these medications have modest cholesterol-lowering effects when taken alone, but none is as effective as statins are for lowering cholesterol and preventing atherosclerosis. Statins go right to the source of the problem— genetic defects in LDL receptor activity—and correct it. They are the mainstay of pharmaceutical treatment.

To put the safety of statins in perspective, you're much more likely to experience serious side effects from aspirin. If you're at risk for atherosclerosis and you're not taking a statin, you are missing out on one of modern medicine's most effective medications.

KEY IDEAS FOR TAKEOUT

- Statins are among the safest and easiest-to-take modern medications.

- The only serious side effect is muscle damage, which occurs in less than half a percent of patients. This usually resolves within a week or two of stopping the medication. Rarely, this reaction causes kidney failure.

- Minor muscle aches occur in 2 to 3 percent of patients. If you experience side effects, talk to your doctor; there are usually ways to circumvent side effects.

CHAPTER 20

Is Daily Aspirin Therapy for You?

"Take two aspirin and call me in the morning." Supposedly, that's what doctors say when they have nothing better to offer. Aspirin has thus become a cliché for a feeble but innocuous nostrum. But aspirin is neither weak nor harmless. It has profound effects on blood clotting. A single aspirin tablet can inhibit coagulation for up to two weeks. Daily aspirin can reduce the risk of heart attack by as much as 40 percent—more than cardiac surgery, angioplasty, or any drug except a statin (see chapters 18 and 19). It prevents heart attacks not only in people with known artery disease, but also in those who only have risk factors like high blood cholesterol, diabetes, smoking, or high blood pressure.

SO, WHAT'S THE DOWNSIDE?

Aspirin also has serious side effects. You may worry more about medications with less familiar names, but, in fact, the most dangerous pill you're likely to take is aspirin.

Aspirin's most troublesome complication is stomach bleeding. Gastrointestinal hemorrhage from aspirin and other drugs of its type—collectively called anti-inflammatory drugs—is by far the number-one cause of medication-related deaths in the United States. To put the magnitude of this problem in perspective, consider that in 1997, 15,800 Americans died of AIDS, while 15,200 died of fatal gastrointestinal bleeding from anti-inflammatory drugs.

Aspirin also increases the risk of certain kinds of strokes, those caused by bleeding in the brain. However, it helps avert strokes caused by blood clots, so the stroke preventive benefits usually outweigh the risks. Nevertheless, because most bleeding-type strokes occur in patients with poorly controlled high blood pressure, you should be sure your blood pressure is properly treated before starting daily aspirin.

You're probably thinking, "I've taken aspirin before, and it didn't seem to bother me." An occasional aspirin is one thing; taking it every day over a long period of time is another. Aspirin can gradually erode the stomach lining. It may not cause trouble at first, but you may experience serious side effects after several months.

You need to take this decision seriously. It's a good idea

to learn how the drug works and how to maximize its bene-fits, minimize its risks, and deal with its side effects.

UNDERSTANDING HOW ASPIRIN WORKS

Aspirin doesn't prevent cholesterol from infiltrating arteries and forming plaques. Nor does it prevent plaques from rup-turing. It prevents artery blockage because it reduces the size of the clots that result from plaque rupture.

Aspirin works by inhibiting the action of platelets, tiny cells in your blood that protect against bleeding. Normally, when something pierces or tears an artery lining, platelets adhere to the edges of the hole, cling together, and form a clot to stop the bleeding. Platelets respond the same way to tears in the artery lining caused by ruptured plaques. In an attempt to repair the damage, they form a clot on the plaque. However, although nature's intent is to form a patch, some-times the clump gets so big it completely blocks blood flow through the artery. Here is where aspirin comes in.

The first platelets to arrive at an area of blood vessel dam-age release a potent chemical called *thromboxane*, which attracts other platelets to the site and causes them to stick together. Aspirin deactivates the enzyme that produces thromboxane. By interfering with platelet clumping, it helps prevent small clots from becoming large clots.

Remarkably, while aspirin's anti-inflammatory and painkilling effects last only a few hours, its effect on platelets continues for *weeks*. Unlike other cells in the body, platelets cannot regenerate thromboxane. Aspirin inhibits platelets' ability to clot for the several-week duration of their lifespan in the bloodstream.

Although other anti-inflammatory drugs have transient effects on platelet clumping, aspirin is the only one that permanently deactivates thromboxane.

Because aspirin doesn't alter the underlying process of cholesterol accumulation and plaque buildup, its protective benefits against artery blockage disappear when the effects on the platelets wear off. Thus, if you take aspirin for a few months and stop, that ends your protection against heart attacks or strokes.

DECIDING WHETHER YOU SHOULD TAKE DAILY ASPIRIN

Despite its usefulness, daily aspirin is not for everyone. You should take it only if the benefits outweigh the risks—if the possibility of preventing a heart attack is greater than the chances of life-threatening stomach bleeding or brain hemorrhage. To help doctors decide who should take daily aspirin, heart associations have established the following guidelines based on research on thousands of patients:

▸ Consider taking daily aspirin if you have evidence of blood-vessel disease: angina, heart attack, stroke, or a test showing artery disease.

▸ Consider taking daily aspirin if you are fifty or older and have two or more of the following risk factors:
  • High LDL
  • Low HDL
  • Type 2 diabetes
  • Current cigarette smoking

- Heart attack in an immediate family member
- High blood pressure

▸ You should not take daily aspirin if you're not at higher-than-average risk of having a heart attack. The chance of serious side effects outweighs the odds of aspirin helping you. If you have only high blood cholesterol and no other risk factors, the risk exceeds the benefit.

If you have tried taking daily aspirin and have had side effects, talk to your physician about alternative treatments or ways to reduce side effects.

TIPS FOR TAKING DAILY ASPIRIN

Doctors have known about the painkilling properties of salicylic acid, the active ingredient of aspirin, since the early 1800s, but stomach irritation and nausea limited its usefulness. Only when Bayer chemists reworked it into a less irritating compound did it become popular. Nevertheless, stomach pain, nausea, aggravation of heartburn, and gastrointestinal bleeding remain troublesome side effects.

Here are some ways to reduce the risk of side effects:

1. Take a children's-strength aspirin—no more. Fortunately, the dose of aspirin needed to inhibit platelets is much less than that required for relief of headache or joint pains. The standard pain-relieving dose is 640 milligrams, but to prevent heart attacks, you need only 81 milligrams a day, the amount in a children's-strength aspirin. In fact, there are diminishing returns to taking higher doses. Taking more

than 160 milligrams per day causes more side effects and actually inhibits clotting *less* than the smaller doses.

2. Take a coated tablet. The main reason aspirin causes stomach irritation and bleeding is that after it enters the bloodstream, it circulates back to the wall of the stomach, where it inhibits enzymes that protect the stomach lining. Nevertheless, there is some direct irritation, so some manufacturers put protective coatings on their tablets to keep aspirin from contacting the stomach lining. This reduces irritation and bleeding slightly, but doesn't prevent such side effects completely. However, if you're going to take aspirin for more than a few days, take the coated kind.

3. Take daily aspirin upon awakening. If you lie down after taking aspirin, it may back up into your lower esophagus and cause heartburn, especially if you have problems with stomach acid reflux. I have seen heartburn sufferers who take only two anti-inflammatory pills per month experience relief when they abstained completely from the drugs.

4. If you take another anti-inflammatory drug, such as ibuprofen or naproxen, hold off taking your daily aspirin for two hours. Taking another anti-inflammatory drug immediately before taking aspirin can interfere with aspirin's anticlotting effects. If you take the aspirin first, wait thirty minutes before taking another antiinflammatory pill.

DEALING WITH SIDE EFFECTS

Aspirin-induced stomach irritation typically causes a

burning discomfort in the pit of the abdomen or beneath the lower part of the breastbone, often accompanied by nausea. These symptoms are usually worse in the morning and subside later in the day. Antacid medication often provides temporary relief. Because heart trouble can cause pain in the same area, check with your doctor. Don't just assume that aspirin is causing these symptoms.

People can often take aspirin without side effects for long periods until something else adds to the stomach irritation. Here are some of the common culprits:

▸ Other anti-inflammatory, anti-arthritis drugs
▸ Anti-osteoporosis drugs (alendronate and risedronate)
▸ Large doses of vitamin C
▸ Certain antibiotics
▸ Nicotine
▸ Alcohol

Dealing with Stomach Irritation

Aspirin-induced abdominal pain or nausea will usually go away in a few days if you give your stomach a two- or three-day vacation from the drug. It's generally safe to stop taking aspirin for that long, because the anticlotting effect lasts for more than a week. Acid-blocking medication, such as omeprazole (Prilosec), will speed relief.

If you have a condition that causes vomiting for more than twenty-four hours, you should stop taking aspirin and contact your doctor. Stomach irritation caused by intestinal flu or food poisoning is usually worse if you're taking aspirin. Such illnesses also can trigger stomach bleeding. (One of the few medication-related deaths I have seen among my patients was that of an elderly woman who took several doses of full-strength aspirin in an attempt to treat intestinal flu.)

You should be aware that aspirin is notorious for damaging the stomach lining and causing dangerous bleeding *without* pain. The only sign of bleeding might be black or bloody stools, weakness, or fainting.

It takes a lot of blood to cause stools to change color, so mild stomach bleeding often goes unnoticed. Sometimes, the only way it can be detected is through blood or stool tests. When patients taking aspirin show signs of internal bleeding, doctors are obliged *not* to assume that aspirin is the culprit. Because cancer and ulcers can trigger similar bleeding, doctors often recommend further tests such as barium enema and colonoscopy. One of the disadvantages of taking aspirin is the likelihood that you may require tests to exclude other causes of intestinal bleeding.

If side effects keep recurring, consider taking a daily antacid such as omeprazole (Prilosec). This will often prevent side effects.

SAMPLING ALTERNATIVES TO ASPIRIN

Pharmaceutical companies have developed medications that can substitute for aspirin or, when taken in addition to aspirin, can improve its effectiveness. One such drug, clopidogrel (Plavix), does as well at preventing heart attacks as aspirin does, with less stomach irritation, and when it is combined with aspirin, it slightly improves aspirin's heart-attack-preventive effects. However, clopidogrel is expensive and has other side effects. Most cardiologists I know think that it provides too little additional benefit and is too expensive to be used in situations in which aspirin alone should be

Aspirin's Fickle Ways

Individuals vary widely in their susceptibility to aspirin's side effects. You may know people who take large amounts of aspirin or other anti-inflammatory drugs without apparent problems. The likelihood of complications increases with age. You might have taken aspirin, ibuprofen, or naproxen for years without problems, and then you start experiencing mysterious stomach pains or nausea without suspecting that the drug is causing them.

Because food neutralizes stomach acid, it can temporarily relieve the discomfort of stomach irritation. The only symptom of aspirin-induced gastritis might be a barely perceptible ache in the pit of your abdomen after you haven't eaten for several hours. Sometimes, this discomfort feels like hunger pangs and increases the urge to eat. Many nutritionists suggest that dieters avoid stomach-irritating medications such as aspirin to prevent overeating.

You should be vigilant when taking aspirin and try to distinguish feelings of hunger from actual pain. If your hunger pangs are truly painful, treat them as aspirin-induced gastritis.

effective. Whether clopidogrel deserves its nickname "Super Aspirin" is yet to be determined.

USING THE DYNAMIC DUO

A daily aspirin and a statin type of cholesterol-lowering medication are a potent combination for preventing heart attacks and strokes. Statins shrink atherosclerotic plaques and prevent them from rupturing; aspirin prevents blockage-producing clots from forming when rupture does occur.

When I started practicing cardiology twenty-five years ago, I was often called to the hospital at all hours of the day or night to take care of patients with heart attacks. Life is easier now. I go for months without having to make an emergency trip to the hospital. My patients rarely have heart attacks, and I attribute this to the use of statins and aspirin.

The existence of medication that prevents heart attacks can be immensely helpful to you in another way. It can allow you to focus your effort on other things. If you're overweight or have signs of insulin resistance but also have a high LDL level, you can take medication to address the cholesterol problem and direct your dietary and exercise efforts in ways that will benefit the carbohydrate side of your metabolism.

KEY IDEAS FOR TAKEOUT

- One baby aspirin a day can reduce your risk of heart attack by as much as 40 percent—more than cardiac surgery, angioplasty, or any drug except statins can.

- Daily aspirin can cause serious side effects. The most common serious complication of aspirin is stomach bleeding.

- If you have no risk factors for blood-vessel disease, you should not take daily aspirin. The chances of being harmed by its side effects outweigh the potential benefits of taking it.

- Aspirin commonly causes stomach pain and nausea.

- The combination of daily aspirin and cholesterol-lowering medication is an especially potent duo for preventing heart attacks and strokes.

- This chapter provides heart association guidelines for deciding if you should take daily aspirin.

CHAPTER 21

Seeing the Pieces of the Puzzle Come Together

Pat answers to health problems would work if all bodies responded the same way, but the reality is different. Some of us have trouble handling carbohydrates, some of us have genetic defects in our cholesterol-metabolizing enzymes, some of us have both, and some, neither.

MESHING YOUR PERSONAL HEALTH INFO WITH THE NEW NUTRITION

By using the New Low-Carb Way—analyzing your body chemistry and tailoring diet, exercise, and medication to your own metabolism—you can walk away with a coherent regimen that will help you lower your cholesterol, attain a healthy body weight, and prevent diabetes.

You grow your understanding of your metabolism—how well your body removes cholesterol from your blood and how well it handles carbohydrates—and you use that, along with information from a simple blood test, body measurements, and your medical history, to come up with a plan, figuring into the mix the problems you should regard as immediate threats and ones that are dangerous only in the long run.

DOING THE RIGHT THING(S)

By assessing your body's capacity to clear cholesterol from the bloodstream and its ability to handle carbohydrates, you can tell what part of your body chemistry you need to concentrate on.

What you do about the cholesterol side of your metabolism has to fit with your carbohydrate side. Addressing one side will inevitably drain resources from the other. If you cut fat from your diet, you need to make sure you don't aggravate insulin resistance and gain weight by eating more refined carbohydrates. On the other hand, if you take cholesterol-lowering medication, you can focus your effort on cutting refined carbohydrates.

You have three tools: diet, exercise, and medication. You don't have to limit yourself to one. The surest way to success is an integrated, tailored approach that makes use of all three, if necessary.

Although medications can correct the metabolic defects that raise LDL, to date, there are no good drugs for relieving insulin resistance or losing weight. You have to change your eating and exercise habits.

In the chapters on low-glucose-shock eating and turning on your muscle switch, you learned how to eliminate glucose shocks, improve your body's sensitivity to insulin, and change your fatness set point with as little effort and deprivation as possible. You discovered that a small change in your routine—if it's exactly the right one—can result in dramatic improvement of insulin sensitivity and steady weight loss.

Here is a recap of the three main body-chemistry types and the best approach for each. You may want to review all three so that you know what type you aren't as well as what type you are. In the future, that will help you distinguish advice that pertains to you from recommendations that apply to others.

RECAPPING THE CARBOHYDRATE STRATEGY

This is the approach you take if you are overweight, have insulin resistance or type 2 diabetes, and your LDL is *normal*.

You should focus on the carbohydrate side of your metabolism. Cutting out high-glucose-shock foods and engaging in mild exertion several times a week dramatically improves the body-chemistry disturbances that aggravate these conditions.

If you follow the Carbohydrate Strategy, you'll witness one of the most dramatic effects a lifestyle change can bring. Although you can't measure it easily, insulin resistance subsides immediately. Within a few days, your blood triglyceride level plummets. This will be followed by a steady, two to four-pound-per-month weight loss. Other symptoms—heartburn, fatigue, poor concentration—often improve, too.

If you don't think you're losing weight fast enough, don't restrict your calories further—that will only slow your metabolism and set off a yo-yo dieting cycle. You have one option: intensify your exercise program. Physical activity not only expends calories while you're exercising, it raises the rate you burn them twenty-four hours a day. It helps you lose weight, literally, as you sleep.

REVISITING THE CHOLESTEROL STRATEGY

Follow this strategy if your LDL is high and you are *not* overweight and you *do not* have insulin resistance or diabetes. To lower your blood levels of bad cholesterol, you should try reducing your intake of saturated fat and replacing the lost calories with complex carbohydrates and unsaturated fat. Remember, though, that the blood-cholesterol response to dietary changes is unpredictable—not nearly as reliable as the response of insulin resistance (see chapter 2) to carbohydrate restriction and exercise. Sometimes LDL levels fall significantly, other times not at all. Sometimes they even go up.

In the end, the average LDL reduction is between 5 and 10 percent, which is usually not low enough to afford adequate protection against artery disease. You should remember that if you have high blood cholesterol, you are dealing with something that could be dangerous and tricky. If your LDL level doesn't drop into the desirable range with a regimen you can live with comfortably, you're probably better off taking cholesterol-lowering medication, which is highly effective, not just for lowering LDL, but for preventing heart attacks and strokes.

If you can't get your LDL down by reducing your saturated fat intake, before going to cholesterol-lowering medication, try reducing your starch and sugar consumption. Occasionally, LDL levels respond favorably to carb restriction even though blood tests and medical history don't suggest insulin resistance or diabetes.

The two situations in which the risk of artery disease is especially high and LDL should be lowered further than usual are: if you already have a blocked artery or if you have type 2 diabetes. The American Heart Association guidelines recommend that if you have either of these conditions, you should get your blood-LDL level below 100. For most patients, that requires cholesterol-lowering medication.

Although people's responses vary, exercise usually doesn't lower blood-LDL levels much. It's certainly not nearly as beneficial to the cholesterol-metabolizing side of your metabolism as it is for the carbohydrate side. Nevertheless, it does raise blood levels of protective cholesterol, stimulate natural anticlotting substances, and improve circulation.

Exercise is especially important if you already have artery disease. It stimulates the growth of new blood vessels into areas served by blocked arteries and helps strengthen and protect the heart.

ONE MORE LOOK AT THE COMBINED STRATEGY

Take this approach if you have problems with both the carbohydrate and the cholesterol sides of your metabolism—that is, if you're overweight, have insulin resistance or type 2 diabetes, and have a *high* blood level of LDL.

The first step is to address the carbohydrate side of your body chemistry by reducing high-glucose-load foods and exercising. If that doesn't bring your LDL down, you have two options: a difficult one that's not very effective or an easy one that is effective. The hard one is trying to control your LDL by reducing your saturated fat and cholesterol intake, in addition to cutting high-glucose-shock foods. The easy, highly effective strategy is to let cholesterol-lowering medication take care of the cholesterol side of your metabolism while you focus your dietary and exercise efforts on the carbohydrate side.

GRABBING HOLD OF THE CONFIDENCE FACTOR

After years of fighting your own body chemistry, you may find it hard to believe there are solutions. You hear so many different claims that you conclude the obvious: the reason there are so many is that none of them works. But millions of man-hours and billions of dollars have been invested in researching these problems in depth, and through the confusing morass of enormous amounts of data, competing viewpoints, irrelevant facts, biases, and commercial interests, answers are beginning to take form.

Similar evolutions of thinking have taken place for other

diseases. For years, doctors were aware of links between smoking and lung cancer, but background noise muddled and obscured them. Scientists still don't know why tobacco causes lung cancer, and there are people who think it doesn't. But at some point, scientists looked objectively at the available information and made a judgment. Cancer isn't destiny. Something causes it. The evidence pointing to tobacco as the culprit was overwhelming, and it was time for action.

We are at a similar stage in our battle against atherosclerosis, obesity, and diabetes. It takes a while to evaluate the validity of each piece of evidence, put it in proper perspective, and see the outlines of answers emerging through the mire of real data, myth, public policy, and profit motive. What you need to do should now be as clear to you as the need to give up smoking is to someone who wants to avoid lung cancer.

THE FACTS

Here are the facts:

▸ Regaining your health isn't complicated. A half-hour walk every other day will help to put your metabolism back on track.

▸ Reducing your intake of flour, potatoes, corn, sugar, and rice is possible.

▸ Facing the fact that you have an inborn error of metabolism that keeps your body from removing cholesterol efficiently isn't so bad now that medical science has discovered a safe, easy-to-take medication that completely corrects the problem.

In many years of helping people deal with cholesterol, obesity, and diabetes, I have seen what people can and cannot do. The advice I have given you here is something you can do. It's based on the simple and practical assumption that you are more likely to do something if it's easy. If you're realistic about your capabilities and choose the right strategy, you can succeed.

Always keep in mind that when it comes to losing weight, the best weight loss is gentle weight loss. You may not trim fat as quickly as you would like to, but in a month or two—when you feel a loosening of your belt and your blood tests have returned to normal—you will feel great, knowing that you have found a healthier way of living that you can actually sustain for a lifetime. This time when you take off pounds, they are much more likely to stay off!

APPENDIX I
RECOMMENDED READING

WEBSITES

www.newlowcarbway.com Supplement to this book. More tips on low-glucose-shock eating, updated glucose-shock tables, primer on heart disease, instructions for using practice guidelines, advice on choosing a doctor.

www.americanheart.org/profilers An interactive tool provided by the American Heart Association for helping people make informed decisions about high blood cholesterol, high blood pressure, and several heart conditions.

www.atkins.com Hundreds of recipes for low-carbohydrate dishes. (All are low-glucose shock.)

www.sugarbusters.com More delicious, low-glucose-shock dishes from New Orleans.

BOOKS

Dr. Atkins' New Carbohydrate Gram Counter (M. Evans)

Dr. Atkins' New Diet Cookbook (M. Evans)

Dr. Atkins' Quick & Easy New Diet Cookbook (Fireside). Hundreds of recipes for low-carbohydrate dishes. (All are low glucose shock.)

Atkins' Best Recipes (Roundtable). Some favorite recipes from Atkins' cookbooks, with photographs.

Sugar Busters! Quick & Easy Cookbook (Ballantine). Delicious low-glucose-shock dishes from New Orleans.

Betty Crocker's Low-Fat, Low-Cholesterol Cooking Today (Betty Crocker). Proven favorites for those on low-fat, low-cholesterol diets.

Fantastic Food with Splenda (M. Evans)

Fitness Walking for Dummies by Liz Neporent (For Dummies). Comprehensive guide to walking for fitness. Includes information on shoes, gadgets, techniques, and health benefits.

Weight Training for Beginners by Tony Gallagher (HarperResource). A good way to start a muscle-building program.

Essentials of Exercise Physiology by William McArdle, Frank Katch, and Victor Katch (Lippincott, Williams, & Wilkins). For those who want to deepen their knowledge of metabolism, diet, and exercise. Written for nondoctors.

Unbelievable Desserts with Splenda (M. Evans)

APPENDIX 2
GLUCOSE-SHOCK
RATINGS OF FOODS

Food Item	Description	Glycemic Index	Available Carboyhydrate (percent)	Typical American Serving	Glucose Shock Rating
LAB STANDARD					
White bread	30 grams ½" slice	100	47	1¹⁄₁₈" oz	100
BAKED GOODS					
Oatmeal cookie	1 medium	77	68	1 oz	102
Apple muffin (sugarless)	2½" diameter	69	32	2½ oz	107
Cookie (average all types)	1 medium	84	64	1 oz	114
Croissant	1 medium	96	46	1½ oz	127
Crumpet	1 medium	69	38	2 oz	148
Bran muffin	2½" diameter	85	42	2 oz	149
Pastry	Average serving	84	46	2 oz	149
Chocolate Cake	1 slice (4" × 3" × 1")	54	47	3 oz	154
Vanilla wafers	4 wafers	110	72	1 oz	159

Food Item	Description	Glycemic Index	Available Carbohydrate (percent)	Typical American Serving	Glucose Shock Rating
Graham Cracker	1 rectangle	106	72	1 oz	159
Blueberry muffin	2½" diameter	84	51	2 oz	169
Pita bread	1 medium	82	57	2 oz	189
Carrot cake	1 square (3" × 3" × ½")	88	56	2 oz	199
Carrot muffin	2½" diameter	88	56	2 oz	199
Waffle	7" diameter	109	37	2½ oz	203
Doughnut	1 medium	108	49	2 oz	205
Cupcake	2½" diameter	104	68	1½ oz	213
Angel food cake	1 slice (4" × 4" × 1")	95	58	2 oz	216
English muffin	1 medium	109	47	2 oz	224
Pound cake	1 slice (4" × 4" × 1")	77	53	3 oz	241
Corn muffin	2½" diameter	146	51	2 oz	299
Pancake	5" diameter	96	73	2½ oz	346
ALCOHOLIC BEVERAGES					
Spirits	1½ oz	Less than 15		1½ oz	Less than 15
Red wine	6 oz	Less than 15		6 oz	Less than 15
White wine	6 oz	Less than 15		6 oz	Less than 15
NONALCHOHOLIC BEVERAGES					
Tomato Juice	6 oz	54	4	6 oz	27
Carrot juice	6 oz	61	12	6 oz	68
Grapefruit juice (unsweetened)	6 oz	69	9	6 oz	75
Apple juice (unsweetened)	6 oz	57	12	6 oz	82
Orange Juice	6 oz	71	10	6 oz	89
Cranberry juice	6 oz	80	12	6 oz	109
Pineapple juice	6 oz	66	14	6 oz	109
Chocolate milk	8 oz	49	10	8 oz	82
Raspberry smoothie	8 oz	48	16	8 oz	127
Coca-Cola	12 oz	90	10	12 oz	218
Gatorade	20 oz	111	6	20 oz	273
Orange soda	8 oz	97	14	12 oz	314
BREADS AND ROLLS					
Tortilla (wheat)	1 medium	43	52	1¾ oz	64
Pizza crust	1 slice	43	22	3½ oz	70
Tortilla (corn)	1 medium	74	48	1¼ oz	87
White bread	1 slice	100	47	1¼ oz	107
Whole-meal rye bread	⅜" slice	97	40	2 oz	114
Sourdough bread	⅜" slice	77	47	1½ oz	114

Food Item	Description	Glycemic Index	Available Carboyhydrate (percent)	Typical American Serving	Glucose Shock Rating
Oat bran bread	⅜" slice	68	60	1½ oz	128
Whole wheat bread	1 slice ½" thick	101	43	1½ oz	129
Light rye bread	⅜" slice	97	47	1½ oz	142
Banana bread (sugarless)	1 slice (4" X 4" X 1")	79	48	3 oz	170
80% whole-kernel oat bread	⅜" slice	93	63	1½ oz	170
Pita bread	8" diameter	82	57	2 oz	189
Hamburger bun	Top & bottom (5" diameter)	87	50	2½ oz	213
80% whole-kernel wheat bread	⅜" slice	74	67	2¼ oz	213
French bread	1 slice (½" thick)	136	50	2 oz	284
Bagel	1 medium	103	50	3⅓ oz	340
BREAKFAST CEREALS					
All-Bran	½ cup	54	77	1 oz	85
Muesli	1 cup	69	53	1 oz	95
Special K	1 cup	98	70	1 oz	133
Cheerios	1 cup	106	40	1 oz	142
Shredded wheat	1 cup	107	67	1 oz	142
Grape-Nuts	1 cup	102	70	1 oz	142
Puffed wheat	1 cup	105	70	1 oz	151
Instant oatmeal (cooked)	1 cup	94	10	8 oz	154
Cream of Wheat (cooked)	1 cup	94	10	8 oz	154
Total	1 cup	109	73	1 oz	161
Corn flakes	1 cup	116	77	1 oz	199
Rice Krispies	1 cup	117	87	1 oz	208
Rice Chex	1 cup	127	87	1 oz	218
Raisin Bran	1 cup	87	63	2 oz	227
CANDY					
Life Saver	1 piece	100	100	⅒ oz	20
Peanut M&Ms	1 snack-size package	47	57	¾ oz	43
White chocolate	2 squares (1" X 1" X ¼")	63	44	⅔ oz	49
Chocolate	2 1" X 1" squares (¼" thick)	61	44	1 oz	68
Snickers bar	1 regular-size bar	97	57	2 oz	218
Jelly beans	⅓ cup	112	93	1½ oz	312
CHIPS AND CRACKERS					
Potato chips	Small bag	77	42	1 oz	62
Corn chips	Small bag	90	52	1 oz	97

Food Item	Description	Glycemic Index	Available Carbohydrate (percent)	Typical American Serving	Glucose Shock Rating
Popcorn	4 cups	103	55	1 oz	114
Rye crisps	1 rectangle	91	64	1 oz	125
Wheat thins	4 small	96	68	1 oz	136
Soda cracker	2 regular	106	68	1 oz	136
Pretzels	Small bag	119	67	1 oz	151
DAIRY PRODUCTS					
Cheese	2" X 2" X 1" slice	Less than 15	0	2 oz	Less than 15
Butter	1 tablespoon	Less than 15	0	¼ oz	Less than 15
Margarine	Typical serving	Less than 15	0	¼ oz	Less than 15
Sour cream	Typical serving	Less than 15	0	2 oz	Less than 15
Yogurt plain, unsweetened	½ cup	51	5	4 oz	17
Yogurt (low-fat, sweetened)	½ cup	47	16	4 oz	57
Chocolate milk (low fat)	8 oz	49	10	8 oz	82
Milk (whole)	8 oz	38	5	8 oz	27
Vanilla ice cream (high fat)	½ cup	54	18		68
Vanilla ice cream (low fat)	½ cup	67	20	4 oz	114
Frozen tofu	½ cup	164	30	4 oz	379
FRUIT					
Strawberries	1 cup	57	3	5½ oz	13
Apricot	1 medium	82	8	2 oz	24
Grapefruit	1 half	36	9	4½ oz	32
Plum	1 medium	55	10	3 oz	36
Kiwifruit	1 medium	75	10	3 oz	43
Peach	1 medium	60	9	4 oz	47
Grapes	1 cup (40 grapes)	66	15	2½ oz	47
Pineapple	1 slice (¾", 3½" wide)	59	11	3 oz	50
Watermelon	1 cup cubed	103	5	5½ oz	52
Pear	1 medium	54	9	6 oz	57
Mango	½ cup	73	14	3 oz	57
Orange	1 medium	60	9	6 oz	71
Apple	1 medium	52	13	5½ oz	78
Banana	1 medium	74	17	3¾ oz	85
Raisins	2 tablespoons	91	73	1 oz	133
Figs	3 medium	87	43	2 oz	151
Dates	5 medium	147	67	1½ oz	298

Glucose Shock Ratings of Foods

Food Item	Description	Glycemic Index	Available Carbohydrate (percent)	Typical American Serving	Glucose Shock Rating
MEAT					
Beef	10-oz steak	Less than 15		10 oz	Less than 15
Pork	2 5-oz chops	Less than 15		10 oz	Less than 15
Chicken	1 breast	Less than 15		10 oz	Less than 15
Fish	8-oz fillet	Less than 15		8 oz	Less than 15
Lamb	3 4-oz chops	Less than 15		12 oz	
NUTS					
Peanuts	¼ cup	21	8	1¼ oz	7
Cashews	¼ cup	31	26	1¼ oz	21
PASTA					
Asian bean noodles	1 cup	47	25	5 oz	118
Whole meal spaghetti	1 cup	53	23	5 oz	126
Vermicelli	1 cup	50	24	5 oz	126
Spaghetti (boiled 5 min)	1 cup	54	27	5 oz	142
Spaghetti (boiled 10–15 min)	1 cup	64	27	5 oz	166
Spaghetti (boiled 20 min)	1 cup	87	24	5 oz	213
Fettucine	1 cup	57	23	5 oz	142
Noodles (Instant 1–2 min)	1 cup	67	22	5 oz	150
			25		
Capellini	1 cup	64	25	5 oz	158
Linguine	1 cup	74	25	5 oz	181
Macaroni	1 cup	67	28	5 oz	181
Rice noodles	1 cup	87	22	5 oz	181
Macaroni and cheese (boxed)	1 cup	92	28	5 oz	252
Gnocchi	1 cup	97	27	5 oz	260
SOUPS					
Tomato soup	1 cup	54	7	8 oz	55
Minestrone	1 cup	56	7	8 oz	64
Lentil soup	1 cup	63	8	8 oz	82
Split pea soup	1 cup	86	11	8 oz	145
Black bean soup	1 cup	92	11	8 oz	154
SWEETENERS					
Artificial Sweeteners	1 teaspoon	Less than 15		⅙ oz	Less than 15
Honey	1 teaspoon	78	72	⅙ oz	16
Table sugar	1 round teaspoon	97	100	⅙ oz	28
Syrup	¼ cup	97		2 oz	364

Food Item	Description	Glycemic Index	Available Carboyhydrate (percent)	Typical American Serving	Glucose Shock Rating
VEGETABLES					
Lettuce	1 cup	Less than 15		2½ oz	Less than 15
Spinach	1 cup	Less than 15		2½ oz	Less than 15
Cucumber	1 cup	Less than 15		6 oz	Less than 15
Mushrooms	½ cup	Less than 15		2 oz	Less than 15
Asparagus	4 spears	Less than 15		3 oz	Less than 15
Peppers	½ medium	Less than 15		2 oz	Less than 15
Broccoli	½ cup	Less than 15		1½ oz	Less than 15
Carrot (raw)	1 medium (7½" length)	23	10	3 oz	11
Carrot (boiled)	⅔ cup	70	6	3 oz	21
Tomato	1 medium	Less than 15		5 oz	Less than 15
Peas	¼ cup	68	9	1½ oz	16
Lentils	½ cup	42	11	3½ oz	33
Butter beans	½ cup	44	13	3 oz	34
Kidney beans	½ cup	39	17	3 oz	40
Navy beans	½ cup	69	10	3 oz	40
Garbanzo beans	½ cup	39	20	3 oz	45
Lima beans	½ cup	46	12	3 oz	57
Pinto beans	½ cup	55	17	3 oz	57
Black-eyed peas	½ cup	59	20	3 oz	74
Yam	½ cup	53	24	5 oz	123
Potato (instant mashed)	¾ cup	122	13	5 oz	161
Potato (baked)	1 medium	121	20	5 oz	246
Sweet potato	1 cup	87	19	5 oz	161
Corn on the cob	1 ear	78	21	5⅓ oz	171
Couscous	½ cup	93	23	4 oz	174
Rice cakes	1 medium	110	84	1 oz	193
French fries	Medium serving (McDonald's)	107	19	5¼ oz	219
Brown rice	1 cup	79	22	6½ oz	222
Basmati rice	1 cup	83	25	6½ oz	271
White rice	1 cup	91	24	6½ oz	283
MISCELLANEOUS					
Eggs	Typical serving	Less than 15		1½ oz	Less than 15
Salad dressing	Typical serving	Less than 15		2 oz	Less than 15

APPENDIX 3
MENUS
DAY I

LOW-GLUCOSE-SHOCK PATTERN		Glucose Shock Rating	TYPICAL PATTERN		Glucose Shock Rating
Breakfast:	Grapefruit	32	**Breakfast:**	Orange juice	68
	Bacon	0		Cornflakes, no sugar	199
	Eggs	0		Milk	27
	Coffee	0		Coffee	0
	1/2 teaspoon sugar	14			
Snack:	Latte	27	**Snack:**	Coffee	0
	Apple	78		Doughnut	205
Lunch:	Chicken Caeser Salad	0	**Lunch:**	Turkey sandwich	260
	Milk	27		Potato chips	77
				Coca-Cola	218
Snack:	Mixed nuts	7	**Snack:**	Corn chips	97
Dinner	Green salad	0	**Dinner**	Caeser salad	0
	New York steak	0		Spaghetti, 2 cups	332
	Mushrooms	0		French bread	284
	Asparagus	0		Butter	0
	1/3 baked potato	82		Red wine	0
	Butter	0			
	Sour cream	0			
	Red wine	0			
Dessert:	Dark Chocolate	68	**Dessert:**	Cookie	114
TOTAL GLUCOSE-SHOCK RATING: 335			**TOTAL GLUCOSE-SHOCK RATING: 1,881**		

DAY 2

LOW-GLUCOSE-SHOCK PATTERN		Glucose Shock Rating	TYPICAL PATTERN		Glucose Shock Rating
Breakfast:	Orange juice	68	**Breakfast:**	Two pancakes	692
	Ham and cheese omelet	0		Milk	27
				Black coffee	0
	Coffee,	0			
	½ teaspoon sugar	14			
Snack:	Latte	27	**Snack:**	Black coffee	0
	Peach	47		Banana	85
Lunch:	Tomato and mozzarella cheese	0	**Lunch:**	Tomato soup	55
	Minestrone	64		Soda crackers, 4	272
				Milk	27
Snack:	Beef jerky	0	**Snack:**	Pretzels	97
	Milk	27		Coca-Cola	218
Dinner	Spinach and gorgonzola salad	0	**Dinner**	Green salad	0
	Baked chicken, 2 pieces	0		Salmon	0
	Asparagus	0		Mashed potatoes	161
	Brown rice, ⅓ cup	74		Corn on the cob	171
	Milk	27		Cranberry juice	109
Dessert:	Peanut M&Ms	43	**Dessert:**	Cupcake	213
TOTAL GLUCOSE-SHOCK RATING: 391			**TOTAL GLUCOSE-SHOCK RATING: 2,127**		

DAY 3

LOW-GLUCOSE-SHOCK PATTERN		Glucose Shock Rating	TYPICAL PATTERN		Glucose Shock Rating
Breakfast:	All-Bran cereal	85	**Breakfast:**	Orange juice	68
	Strawberries	6		Bagel	199
	Plain yogurt	13		Coffee	27
	Artificial sweetener	17			
	Coffee	0			
Snack:	Latte	27	**Snack:**	Coffee	0
	Pear	57		Cookie	114
Lunch:	Greek salad	0	**Lunch:**	Tuna-fish sandwich	260
	Lamb	0		Potato chips	62
	Milk	27		Milk	27
Snack:	Cheese	0	**Snack:**	Corn chips	97
	Apple	78		Coca-Cola	218
Dinner	Green salad	0	**Dinner**	Hamburger	213
	Pizza with cheese, sausage, and mushroom topping, ⅔ of crust removed, 3 slices	46		French fries	219
				Coca-Cola	218
Dessert:	Peppermint candy	20	**Dessert:**	Cookie	114
TOTAL GLUCOSE-SHOCK RATING: 376			**TOTAL GLUCOSE-SHOCK RATING: 2,127**		
Three-day total: 1,102			*Three-day total: 5,844*		

ABOUT THE AUTHOR

Preventive cardiologist Rob Thompson, M.D.—board-certified in cardiology and internal medicine—specializes in preventing heart attacks and strokes. For the past twenty-five years, he has practiced internal medicine and preventive cardiology in downtown Seattle, where he has also done research in heart disease. Dr. Thompson graduated from the University of Washington School of Medicine in Seattle in 1971, at a time when the thinking on heart disease was entirely different from where it stands today—a learning curve that he has watched with interest and that he himself has participated in with vigor and enthusiasm.

He did his postgraduate training at the University of Illinois Medical Center in Chicago, and Dr. Thompson was a faculty member at the University of Washington and director of coronary care at Harborview Medical Center in Seattle before entering private practice in 1977. Over the years, he has penned a number of scientific articles for peer-reviewed journals.

Having accumulated the experience and knowledge that equates to amazing insight on weight loss and heart disease, Dr. Thompson sees his latest work—*The New Low-Carb Way of Life*—as an extremely satisfying achievement that amounts to the ultimate patient consultation, in which he is able to share information that will lead readers to greater overall health—a coup that's impossible for any physician in the space of a brief office visit.

In *The New Low-Carb Way of Life*, Dr. Thompson presents a terrific new weight-loss plan that helps you do what was previously unthinkable: customize a low-starch diet to your personal metabolic needs—and also prevent heart disease and diabetes in the process. Designed for the savviest generation of weight-conscious Americans ever, this book has an uplifting message: only certain carbs pack on pounds and clog arteries, and those are easily identifiable white foods, including flour, corn, potatoes, rice, and sugar.

Dr. Thompson promises that you can attain peak health without having to abandon your current way of living. You simply make a few small changes in your lifestyle—ones that won't make you feel deprived, leave you hungry, or wear you out. You can use the New Low-Carb Way to shed unwanted pounds, improve your overall health, and feel newly empowered and confident.

INDEX

Index

Index